Journal of Health Politics, Policy and Law

Volume 45, Number 4, August 2020
Published by Duke University Press

Contents

Introduction:
The ACA at 10

Jonathan Oberlander
University of North Carolina at Chapel Hill

The study of health care politics in the United States has long been pre-occupied with failure. During the twentieth century, efforts to enact national health insurance repeatedly ended in defeat. Medicare and Medicaid offered an important exception to the norm, though their passage in 1965 presaged not universal health insurance but, rather, further incremental extensions of government coverage to groups, such as children and pregnant women, that commanded political sympathy. From about 1970 to 2010, American health politics operated according to a predictable script: periodic declarations of crisis and calls for urgent action, followed by debate over myriad reform alternatives, all culminating in inaction or incrementalism. As a result, America's uninsured population and health care expenditures climbed upward. The United States became an international outlier in the inequity, insecurity, and expense of its insurance arrangements.

Political scientists offered an array of explanations for the absence of universal insurance in the United States. Fragmented political institutions limited presidents' power, divided reform proponents while giving opponents numerous opportunities to block change, and made it difficult to pass comprehensive legislation through the congressional gauntlet. Influential stakeholder groups used their resources to preserve the profitable status quo for the health care industry and resist measures that threatened their income. Americans' ambivalence about government and fear of anything labeled *socialism* made it hard for reformers to attract and sustain public

Journal of Health Politics, Policy and Law, Vol. 45, No. 4, August 2020
DOI 10.1215/03616878-8255409   © 2020 by Duke University Press

support and helped antireform groups scare the public about the allegedly dire consequences of reform ("socialized medicine").

The proposals to enact new government insurance programs that overcame these obstacles to become law did so by embracing incrementalism and compromising with stakeholder interests. The price for legislative success was limiting public coverage to select populations, forgoing universal coverage, building on existing arrangements, and avoiding cost containment. As spending consequently rose, so too did the price of paying for universal coverage. And the patchwork insurance nonsystem that the United States did establish—comprising Medicare, Medicaid, employer-sponsored insurance, and more—created yet another barrier to reform. Americans were divided into different programs that developed their own constituencies and stakeholders, thereby generating a politics of inertia among the already insured and hindering efforts to disrupt those arrangements or enact a single national health plan that would eliminate the fragmentation.

Many analysts wondered if the United States could ever circumvent these daunting barriers to pass comprehensive reform. The enactment of the Affordable Care Act (ACA) in 2010 was thus a landmark political and policy achievement. Its passage, which was enabled partly by Democrats securing the only filibuster-proof supermajority in the Senate attained by either party between 1980 and 2020, contravened assumptions about American health care politics and the intransigence of the status quo. Judged against prior programs and the typically narrow boundaries of US health policy, the ACA was deeply ambitious, combining a major expansion of access to health insurance with efforts to contain spending and reform health care payment and delivery (including the promotion of accountable care organizations). It moved the United States closer to the norm that all persons should have access to insurance and vastly expanded the federal government's role in regulating health markets.

During its first decade, the ACA has transformed American health care, creating a more equitable, accessible, and (for some) affordable insurance system. About 20 million Americans have gained health insurance. Insurers can no longer discriminate against persons on the basis of health status and preexisting conditions. The law's Medicaid expansion and subsidies to buy private insurance have enabled millions of Americans with modest means to obtain coverage. Moreover, national health spending has grown at a much more moderate rate than predicted at the ACA's enactment.

For all those successes, the ACA has not been without its shortcomings and disappointments. Thirty million persons in the United States still lack health insurance, and the uninsured population, including children, is now growing again. Americans who do not qualify for large subsidies under the ACA struggle to afford coverage in its insurance marketplaces, and many persons with employer-sponsored health plans face high (and rising) deductibles and copayments. ACA policies that were heralded in 2010 as vital cost containment innovations—including the Independent Payment Advisory Board to restrain Medicare spending and the Cadillac tax on high-cost employer plans—have been discarded by Congress, as have taxes on the health insurance and medical device industries. The individual mandate penalty—widely seen a decade ago as essential to the ACA's viability—has been repealed.

The ACA's first decade has generated plenty of surprises. The law has been much more legally vulnerable than anticipated at enactment, saved in a 2012 case only by the deciding vote of Chief Justice John Roberts. The Supreme Court's stunning decision in that same case to make Medicaid expansion effectively optional for states undermined one of the law's foundations, creating a major coverage gap for low-income persons living in states that rejected expansion. Indeed, the ACA's fate in the courts remains unsettled. In the coming years, either the entire law or large portions of it could be scrapped by the Supreme Court in response to an ongoing legal challenge brought by Republican state attorneys general.

Politically, the ACA has shown both remarkable vulnerability and resilience. In Washington, Republicans' opposition to Obamacare has persisted despite the ACA's achievements, widespread benefits, and health industry support. In 2017, the GOP came within a single vote in the Senate of repealing much of the ACA (Republican Senators John McCain, Lisa Murkowski, and Susan Collins, who cast the votes that stopped repeal, joined Chief Justice Roberts as unlikely saviors of the ACA). Even after that failed effort to overturn the law, the Trump administration has attempted to undermine the ACA through administrative actions. Still the law has survived, and amid Republicans' legislative, legal, and administrative assaults it remains mostly intact to date. Medicaid expansion, insurance subsidies, and consumer insurance protections—the ACA's core benefits—are widely popular and reach tens of millions of Americans, making any effort to repeal the ACA politically treacherous.

What lies ahead for the ACA in its second decade? Its future is highly uncertain, contingent on court decisions, electoral results, and political as well as socioeconomic currents that we cannot discern now. Health politics can move in mysterious ways. After all, a decade that began with the ACA preserving private insurance and expanding Medicaid ended with

Republicans attempting to curtail Medicaid eligibility and Democrats proposing Medicare-for-all plans that would displace private insurance. The ACA's enactment was a monumental event; 10 years later, its reverberations continue to reshape US health care policy and politics. The ACA did not end the century-long conflict over health care reform in the United States, but it changed that conflict in ways that will extend far beyond 2020.

The articles in this special issue (which actually spans two issues of *JHPPL*) reflect on the ACA's first decade, evaluating the law's impacts, performance, and evolution from the perspectives of political science, economics, law, health services research, and public health. Authors explore how the ACA has fared compared to original expectations and analyze lessons from the law's implementation and experiences with Medicaid expansion, health insurance marketplaces, choice, and the courts. They illuminate what the ACA tells us about race, policy feedbacks, waivers, federalism, rulemaking, partisanship, and public opinion in American politics, as well as how the ACA looks from a comparative perspective. They examine the ACA in the context of critical health policy issues, including health disparities, health care cost control, and provider consolidation. And they grapple with the ACA's lessons and implications for contemporary reform debates. Taken together, these articles paint a complex portrait of the ACA, its legacies, the state of health care politics, and the enduring challenges in US health policy.

Promise, Performance, and Litigation

Ten Years Later: Reflections on Critics' Worst-Case Scenarios for the Affordable Care Act

Stacey McMorrow
Linda J. Blumberg
John Holahan
Urban Institute

Abstract The primary goals of the Affordable Care Act (ACA) were to increase the availability and affordability of health insurance coverage and thereby improve access to needed health care services. Numerous studies have overwhelmingly confirmed that the law has reduced uninsurance and improved affordability of coverage and care for millions of Americans. Not everyone believed that the ACA would lead to positive outcomes, however. Critics raised numerous concerns in the years leading up to the law's passage and full implementation, including about its consequences for national health spending, labor supply, employer health insurance markets, provider capacity, and overall population health. This article considers five frequently heard worst-case scenarios related to the ACA and provides research evidence that these fears did not come to pass.

Keywords health reform, health insurance coverage, access to care, health care costs

The primary goals of the Affordable Care Act (ACA) were to increase the availability and affordability of health insurance coverage and thereby improve access to needed health care services. The law included numerous provisions aimed at achieving these goals, but the major coverage components were an expansion of Medicaid to adults with incomes at or below 138% of the federal poverty level and the introduction of federal and state-based insurance marketplaces where low- to moderate-income Americans could purchase subsidized private coverage. Among other things, the highly regulated marketplaces increased risk sharing between healthy and sick consumers and eliminated explicit price discrimination based on

Journal of Health Politics, Policy and Law, Vol. 45, No. 4, August 2020
DOI 10.1215/03616878-8255421   © 2020 by Duke University Press

health status. The law also included an extension of dependent coverage to young adults ages 19–25. Each of these provisions was reinforced by a requirement that most Americans have health insurance coverage or pay a penalty (Kaiser Family Foundation 2013).

The implementation of these provisions has evolved considerably in the 10 years since the law was passed. In 2012, the Supreme Court ruled the individual mandate to be constitutional and made adoption of the Medicaid expansion optional for states. As of January 2020, 35 states and the District of Columbia have implemented the ACA Medicaid expansion (Kaiser Family Foundation 2020). Nebraska also passed a ballot initiative supporting expansion but has thus far not implemented expansion, nor is it clear that they will do so. In 2017, the Tax Cuts and Jobs Act eliminated the penalty associated with the requirement to maintain health insurance coverage and thereby effectively eliminated the individual mandate. In addition, the marketplaces have experienced multiple threats to their stability but completed their seventh open enrollment period in December 2019, with 2020 insurer participation up and premiums modestly lower, on average, than in 2019 (Holahan, Wengle, and Elmendorf, 2020).

Numerous studies of the effects of the ACA have overwhelmingly confirmed that the law has reduced uninsurance and improved affordability of coverage and care for millions of Americans (Gruber and Sommers 2019; McMorrow and Polsky 2016). Approximately 20 million people gained health insurance under the law (NCHS 2019), and there is particularly strong evidence that the Medicaid expansion has improved access to and affordability of health care services for low-income adults (Antonisse et al. 2019). Moreover, the Medicaid expansion has improved both hospital and consumer finances (Blavin 2016; Caswell and Waidmann 2019; Hu et al. 2018), and evidence continues to roll in on the law's benefits for specific subgroups of the population, such as racial and ethnic minorities (Wehby and Lyu 2018; Yue, Rasmussen, and Ponce 2018), women and new mothers (Johnston et al. 2018; Daw and Sommers 2019; Gordon et al. 2020), as well as on nonhealth outcomes such as evictions (Zewde et al. 2019).

The mounting evidence on the positive impacts of the ACA stands in stark contrast to some of the predictions from a decade ago suggesting dramatic negative consequences of the law for US health care and the economy. Critics raised numerous concerns in the years leading up to its passage and full implementation, including about its consequences for national health spending, labor supply, employer health insurance markets, provider capacity, and overall population health. Those ideologically opposed to the law voiced these concerns most frequently, but some warnings also came from less partisan sources. In this article, we consider five frequently heard early warnings related to the ACA and provide research evidence that indicates these worst fears did not come to pass. We conclude by discussing where the ACA came up short and consider the lessons learned from a decade of debate, implementation, and evaluation of the law, as well as the implications of these lessons for current debates over appropriate next steps.

Scenario 1: The ACA Will Add to the Deficit and Make National Health Spending Growth Unsustainable

Often one of the biggest points of contention for any major legislative proposal is its cost, and the ACA was no exception. While the official projections by the Congressional Budget Office (CBO) and Joint Committee on Taxation in 2010 and 2011 predicted a net decrease in the deficit as a result of the ACA, they did project increases in federal health spending of $900 billion over 10 years (Elmendorf 2011). Moreover, Centers for Medicare and Medicaid Services (CMS) projections also predicted an overall increase in national health expenditures of $311 billion over 10 years (Foster 2010).

Opponents focused on these projected increases in federal health care spending, ignoring the offsetting spending cuts and tax increases, to claim that the law would add to the federal deficit. In 2011, for example, the Heritage Foundation reported that the marketplace subsidies would "harm the economy by increasing the national deficit" and that "since many of the beneficiaries will be in the upper middle class, Obamacare's subsidies represent a reckless addition to the welfare state" (Winfree 2011).

Despite these criticisms, the ACA included a number of cost-containment provisions, including pilot programs aimed at restructuring the way providers are paid, a tax on overly generous health plans (the so-called Cadillac tax), an Independent Payment Advisory Board intended to rein in Medicare costs, and incentives for nongroup market insurers to compete for enrollees on price. Even so, many observers believed that the increased use of health care services associated with more generous insurance coverage would lead to faster health spending growth and could ultimately crowd out spending on other important services.

Even without the implementation of the Independent Payment Advisory Board or the Cadillac tax, neither of which was ultimately put in place, critics' warnings about the cost of the law were overstated. The ACA did

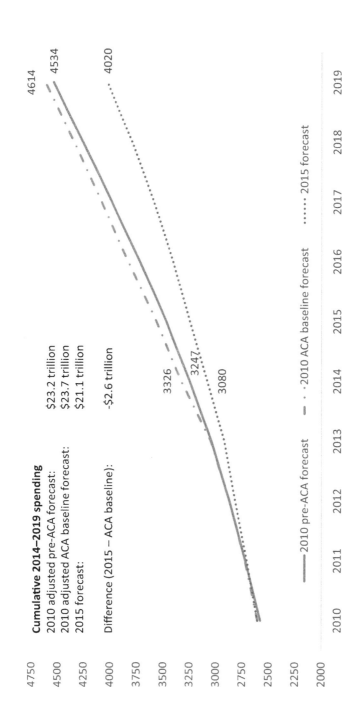

Figure 1 National Health Expenditure Projections ($ Billions), 2010–2019

Notes: Authors' analysis of Centers for Medicare and Medicaid Services national health expenditure projections. Adjusted forecasts reflect alternative scenarios that assume the cuts to physician payments under the sustainable growth rate are replaced with a rate freeze. The 2015 forecast reflects a permanent fix under t1e Medicare Access and CHIP Reauthorization Act (MACRA) of 2015.
Source: Urban Institute (McMorrow and Holahan 2016).

increase federal spending, but by 2017 the CBO and Joint Committee on Taxation estimated that the increases were lower than originally anticipated. For example, at the time the law was passed, the federal cost of the insurance coverage provisions was projected to be $214 billion in 2019, and in March 2017 that projection was revised downward to $148 billion, a reduction of about one-third (CBO 2017). Moreover, national health spending projections have also fallen since the ACA was passed. In 2010, CMS projected that national health spending from 2014 to 2019 would be $23.7 trillion under the ACA (fig. 1). By 2015, however, CMS had revised its projections and estimated that national health spending from 2014 to 2019 would be $21.1 trillion, or $2.6 trillion lower than in the ACA baseline forecast (McMorrow and Holahan 2016).

While some of this reduction in projected spending can be attributed to the Supreme Court decision making the Medicaid expansion optional and lower than anticipated take-up of marketplace coverage, the broader slowdown in health spending growth that began in 2008 and continued well past the end of the recession is a more important factor. The causes of slower health spending growth over this period are not fully understood but likely include the sluggish economic recovery, the rise of high deductible health plans, and strong state Medicaid cost containment efforts. The precise contribution of the ACA to slower spending growth has not been confirmed, but there are reasons to believe it played a role (Cutler and Sahni 2017; Emanuel 2016). Thus, with the federal cost of the law coming in lower than anticipated and no evidence that the ACA led to faster national health spending growth, early fears about rising deficits and insufficient cost containment provisions in the law have largely been alleviated. Real concerns remain, however, about the efficiency of spending in the health care system more generally.

Scenario 2: The ACA Will Suppress Labor Supply

Another widely held concern about the law surrounded its potential effects on the labor market. There were several provisions of the ACA that economists believed could suppress the labor supply. For example, the income eligibility thresholds to qualify for Medicaid expansion and marketplace subsidies create a potential scenario where working less could result in a net benefit for individuals if they became eligible for one of these subsidized programs. Moreover, the employer mandate created incentives for employers to shift their workforce toward greater use of part-time employees, and other tax increases under the law had the potential to suppress productivity.

Early estimates from CBO projected a loss of approximately 800,000 jobs under the ACA, mostly a result of workers choosing to supply less labor, and updated estimates in 2014 nearly tripled that number (CBO 2014b). This became one of the rallying cries of those opposed to the law. A *Forbes* article published in February 2014 concluded: "The bottom line is that the ACA will result in the equivalent of 2.9 million or more fewer working Americans. No amount of hand-waving by the law's proponents can avoid this inconvenient truth" (Conover 2014).

Since then, numerous studies have examined the effects of the dependent coverage expansion and the Medicaid expansion on employment, hours worked, wages, and earnings and have found no evidence to support the predictions described above (Abraham and Royalty 2017; Garrett, Kaestner, and Gangopadhyaya 2017; Kaestner et al. 2017). At least two studies have also considered the effects of marketplace subsidies on labor supply and have found no significant effects (Cucko, Rinz, and Solow 2017; Duggan, Goda, and Jackson 2019). Furthermore, studies examining the potential shift to part-time employment or a trend toward early retirement under the ACA found no evidence to support these claims (Levy, Buchmueller, and Nikpay 2018; Moriya, Selden, and Simon 2016). Overall, the evidence is remarkably consistent across studies looking at the various policy mechanisms and using different outcomes and data sources. While the economic theory supporting a concern about labor supply effects was sound, the evidence suggests that the assumptions used to predict the magnitude of the effects did not adequately reflect the full range of factors beyond health insurance that affect employer and employee preferences.

Scenario 3: The ACA Will Destroy the Employer Health Insurance Market

The components of the law that strengthened and subsidized the private nongroup insurance market contributed to fears about the future of the employer-sponsored health insurance market. When the law was passed in 2010, approximately 57% of nonelderly Americans received health insurance from their employer or that of a family member (fig. 2). The subsidized insurance marketplaces under the ACA presented an alternative to employer coverage and created potential incentives for employers to stop offering coverage to their employees. These incentives were strongest for employers of lower-wage workers who would be eligible for Medicaid or the most generous premium and cost-sharing subsidies under the law. If many employers were to stop offering insurance to their workers, many

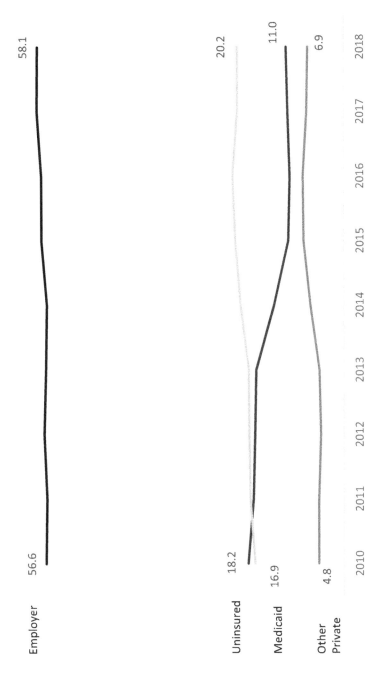

Figure 2 Percent of Nonelderly US population (< 65 Years), by Coverage Type, 2010–2018

Source: National Center for Health Statistics, 2019; National Health Interview Survey: Long-Term Trends in Health Insurance Coverage, 1968–2018.

people would find their source of coverage disrupted and the government cost of the law could increase due to larger numbers of workers and their dependents enrolling in federally subsidized marketplace coverage or Medicaid. As a result, the ACA included a provision to encourage employers to continue to offer coverage. Employers with more than 50 full-time-equivalent employees would pay a $2,000 penalty per worker if they did not offer coverage and one or more employees received a premium subsidy in the marketplace (there is no penalty for workers enrolling in Medicaid). In addition, the ACA did not alter the significant tax advantage of employer-sponsored insurance that predated the law.

The most dramatic predictions suggested extremely widespread dropping of employer coverage. A study by the American Action Forum predicted that as many as 35 million Americans would lose their employer-sponsored coverage, with an associated increase in federal premium subsidies of $1.4 trillion (Holtz-Eakin and Smith 2010). In July 2013, leaders of three major unions seized on this message and sent a letter to Congress claiming that the law's incentives were causing "nightmare scenarios" and would "destroy the very health and wellbeing of our members along with millions of other hardworking Americans" (Gara 2013). Official projections from the CBO (2014a) were much more modest but still predicted employer coverage losses of approximately 6 million people by 2016. In contrast, in 2012, Urban Institute researchers estimated that employer-sponsored insurance would *increase* modestly under the ACA (by less than 3%), due in large part to the individual mandate and persistent tax incentives (Blumberg et al. 2012).

Far from the nightmare scenario predictions, both early and sustained evidence suggests that the employer-sponsored insurance market has remained large and strong under the ACA. Blavin et al. (2015) found no evidence of declines in employer offer, take-up, or coverage rates through 2014, and consistent evidence since then has found stable if not rising rates of employer coverage (Shartzer, Blavin, and Holahan 2018). By 2018, the rate of employer coverage among the nonelderly population was 58.1% compared to 56.6% in 2010 (fig. 2). A strong economy, the law's individual mandate, the continued tax advantage of employer coverage, and turbulence in the marketplaces have likely contributed to the strength and stability of employer coverage in recent years, but there is certainly no evidence to support widespread dropping of coverage under the law.

In addition to fears of employers dropping their health insurance plans, there were also concerns that the Medicaid expansion would cause newly eligible individuals to drop their employer coverage in favor of the more affordable public plan. This "crowd-out" of existing employer coverage is a cause for concern to some because, were it to occur, the federal cost of the law would increase without covering additional individuals. There would be value, however, to low-income people obtaining very comprehensive coverage at little to no cost to the household, since it would improve their health insurance affordability and access to care, potentially improving their downstream health outcomes as well. There is some evidence of displacement of private insurance under the ACA's Medicaid eligibility expansion, but the magnitude of the estimates varies widely, and the results are often imprecise. The smallest estimates indicate virtually no evidence of crowd-out (Frean, Gruber, and Sommers 2017), while the largest indicate significant crowd-out in 2015 that then declined over time (Miller and Wherry 2019). Thus, with no evidence of net declines in employer coverage under the ACA and modest evidence of crowd-out due to the Medicaid expansion, it is clear that the employer-sponsored insurance market remains strong, despite the critics' worst fears.

Scenario 4: Provider Capacity Will Be Insufficient to Meet Demand under the ACA

Despite criticisms on many other fronts, most observers seemed to agree that the ACA would succeed in its effort to increase the number of insured Americans. There was considerable disagreement, however, on whether that coverage would actually provide access to care or improved health. In particular, there was a great deal of concern that the supply and distribution of health care providers would be insufficient to meet the increased demand created by the newly insured. A 2013 *Forbes* article, for example, warned that "America is suffering from a doctor shortage. An influx of millions of new patients into the healthcare system will only exacerbate that shortage—driving up the demand for care without doing anything about its supply" (Pipes 2013). Also in 2013, Joseph Antos argued in this journal that this issue would be particularly problematic for the Medicaid population. Low provider payment rates have historically kept many providers from accepting Medicaid patients, so "putting millions of additional people into a program that has been struggling with access to care for the past forty-five years is likely to result in worsening access for those who are currently enrolled in Medicaid" (Antos 2013).

The ACA included several provisions aimed at shoring up provider access, including a temporary increase in Medicaid fees and increased federal funding for community health centers. A study using a "secret shopper" analysis in 10 states found increased appointment availability for Medicaid patients and stable appointment availability for privately insured patients following the ACA (Polsky et al. 2017). The researchers in this study posed as Medicaid or privately insured patients new to the practice at which they sought an appointment but did not provide further details about their coverage. Moreover, when considering the potential spillover effects of the eligibility expansion on those who were insured prior to the ACA, Carey, Miller, and Wherry (2018) found that Medicare enrollees did not experience any adverse effects of the ACA Medicaid expansion on their access to care. To our knowledge, there is currently no evidence on how the expansion affected access for those who were already enrolled in Medicaid prior to the expansion.

A few studies have found evidence consistent with provider capacity constraints. The same secret shopper study that found increased appointment availability overall found that wait times increased for both Medicaid and privately insured patients (Polsky et al. 2017). Two studies using data from the National Health Interview Survey also found evidence among low-income adults that the Medicaid expansion increased reports of delaying care due to wait time for an appointment and problems finding a provider who could see them (Miller and Wherry 2017; Selden, Lipton, and Decker 2017). These access problems were not trivial in magnitude through 2015, with the share reporting care delays due to appointment wait times increasing by almost one-third (Miller and Wherry 2017), but when data through 2017 were added these access problems had diminished (Miller and Wherry 2019). Moreover, considerable evidence has shown that the ACA Medicaid expansion had a positive effect on having a usual source of care and use of preventive services so any delays or wait times due to capacity constraints did not appear to prevent the law from improving access to and utilization of care for those it targeted (Antonisse et al. 2019; Simon, Soni, and Cawley 2017; Sommers et al. 2015).

Scenario 5: The ACA Will Not Improve, and May Actually Be Harmful to, Population Health

At the end of the day, insurance coverage and even access to and use of health care services do not guarantee good health outcomes, and concerns about the ACA's impact on population health were widespread. Those generally supportive of the law feared that, despite its best intentions, the ACA would not actually move the needle on health outcomes. Some of these concerns were reinforced by the lack of clinical improvement found in a study of the Oregon Health Insurance Experiment (Baicker et al. 2013), as well as growing evidence on the social determinants of health. Recognizing that there are many and varied contributors to good health, even supporters believed that the ACA coverage expansion was necessary but potentially not sufficient to meaningfully improve health status (McMorrow 2010).

In contrast, some of the law's fiercest critics believed that the law would actually harm people's health. Perhaps the most extreme example was Sarah Palin's claim that the law would effectively institute "death panels," or groups of bureaucrats tasked with deciding who was worthy of care (Kessler 2012). But the more insidious claims focused on Medicaid and misinterpreted research evidence to claim that Medicaid was worse than no coverage at all (Carroll and Frakt 2017). Unlike Palin's obviously sensationalist comments, these claims have been made by respected scholars and were used to argue against the ACA more generally (Gottlieb 2011), and then to argue against expanding Medicaid once the Supreme Court made the expansion optional (Antos 2013).

Thus far, the evidence for positive health effects of the ACA Medicaid expansion is weaker than that for coverage or affordability of care, but several important findings have emerged (Allen and Sommers 2019). Several early studies found small or no effects on self-reported general or mental health status (Courtemanche et al. 2018; Miller and Wherry 2017), while others have found improvements in self-reported health and reductions in psychological distress (McMorrow et al. 2017; Simon, Soni, and Cawley 2017). With respect to improved clinical outcomes, researchers found improved blood pressure control among community health center patients, but no improvement for diabetes (Cole et al. 2017). There is also recent evidence that Medicaid expansion improved surgical outcomes for several common conditions, seemingly driven by earlier presentation for care (Loehrer et al. 2018).

When considering mortality, perhaps the ultimate health outcome, there is emerging evidence that the ACA has, in fact, saved lives. Recent work using survey data linked with death records has attributed a 9% reduction in mortality among low-income adults to the Medicaid expansion (Miller et al. 2019), and another study capitalizing on an Internal Revenue Service experiment found that coverage gains for middle-aged adults under the ACA reduced their mortality (Goldin, Lurie, and McCubbin 2019). Thus, despite somewhat inconsistent evidence across a variety of populations and health outcomes, there is little or no evidence to support the claim that the ACA Medicaid expansion has harmed health, and the weight of the evidence appears to indicate health improvements.

Discussion

We have argued above that the ACA failed to live up to its critics' worst fears when it came to cost, labor market effects, the demise of employer coverage, provider capacity constraints, and population health. We must also acknowledge, however, where the ACA underperformed the expectations set by some of its advocates. First, a commonly heard argument for expanding coverage was that it would actually save money by reducing reliance on emergency departments (ED) and improving access to preventive care. While insurance coverage does generally increase use of preventive services, it does not necessarily reduce use of the ED or reduce costs (Russell 2010). Like other services, ED visits typically become less expensive to the consumer after they gain insurance, and when a service becomes less expensive, people tend to use more of it. This pattern was seen following the Oregon health insurance expansion (Taubman et al. 2014), and there is evidence that ED use increased under the ACA Medicaid expansion as well (Garthwaite et al. 2019; Nikpay et al. 2017). This should not be interpreted as a failure of the ACA but, rather, a failure of those promoting an unrealistic outcome.

Second, and more important, despite the ACA's many successes, coverage and care remain unaffordable for too many Americans, particularly many of those who rely on the individual health insurance market. The ACA's marketplaces were intended to provide an affordable option for individuals and families with low to moderate incomes and no access to employer or public coverage. For many marketplace enrollees, this option has improved access to and affordability of care (Kirby and Vistnes 2016; McMorrow et al. 2016). But for those eligible for small premium subsidies or none at all, coverage in the marketplace can be quite expensive (Holahan, Blumberg, and Wengle 2017). Moreover, when individuals seek lower premiums to increase affordability, they generally face high deductibles and other cost-sharing requirements (Gunja et al. 2016). The fundamental driver of high insurance costs is, of course, the high cost of health care itself, so truly delivering on the promise to make health care affordable for all Americans will likely require tackling this head on, as well as funding additional subsidies.

As the 2020 presidential campaign heats up and we begin to debate the merits of various health reform proposals, we should take at least two lessons from over 10 years of ACA debate, implementation, and evaluation. First, one should not take individual projections of costs or other outcomes too literally but, rather, consider the range of estimates and potential outcomes. As we have seen with the ACA, not all predictions will be realized, so it is important not to focus too much attention on any one predicted benefit or cost of a specific proposal. Second, while predictions and projections are an important part of the process of developing and implementing reform proposals, the only way to truly know the effects of a particular policy is to wait for the evidence. And on that front, researchers have delivered a tremendous body of work that should allow anyone interested to form a robust and nuanced opinion of the ACA's successes and failures, and with time, we should expect the same of any future reforms.

▪ ▪ ▪

Stacey McMorrow is a principal research associate in the Health Policy Center at the Urban Institute. She uses quantitative methods to study the factors that affect individual health insurance coverage and access to care, and she has extensive experience analyzing Medicaid eligibility policies and coverage expansions under the Affordable Care Act. She has also worked on topics related to women's health and access to preventive and reproductive health services. SMcMorrow@urban.org

Linda J. Blumberg is an institute fellow in the Health Policy Center at the Urban Institute, which she joined in 1992. She is an expert on private health insurance (employer and nongroup), health care financing, and health system reform. Her recent work includes extensive research related to the Affordable Care Act, including estimating the implications of repeal and replace proposals, interpreting and analyzing the effects of particular policies, and delineating strategies for filling shortcomings in current law.

John Holahan is an institute fellow in the Health Policy Center at the Urban Institute, where he previously served as center director for more than 30 years. His recent work focuses on health reform, the uninsured, health expenditure growth, and developing proposals for health system reform. He examines the coverage, costs, and economic impact of the Affordable Care Act, including the costs of Medicaid expansion as well as the macroeconomic effects of the law.

Acknowledgments

The authors are grateful to all of the researchers who have contributed to such a strong evidence base on the effects of the Affordable Care Act, and to Caroline Elmendorf for excellent research assistance. This work was supported by the Robert Wood Johnson Foundation. The views expressed are those of the authors and should not be attributed to the Urban Institute, its trustees, or its funder.

References

Abraham, Jean, and Anne Beeson Royalty. 2017. "How Has the Affordable Care Act Affected Work and Wages?" Leonard Davis Institute of Health Economics, University of Pennsylvania, Issue Brief, January 19. ldi.upenn.edu/brief/how-has-affordable-care-act-affected-work-and-wages.

Allen, Heidi, and Benjamin D. Sommers. 2019. "Medicaid Expansion and Health: Assessing the Evidence after Five Years." *JAMA* 322, no. 13: 1253–54. doi.org/10.1001/jama.2019.12345.

Antonisse, Larisa, Rachel Garfield, Robin Rudowitz, and Madeline Guth. 2019. "The Effects of Medicaid Expansion under the ACA: Updated Findings from a Literature Review." Kaiser Foundation, August 15. www.kff.org/medicaid/issue-brief/the-effects-of-medicaid-expansion-under-the-aca-updated-findings-from-a-literature-review-august-2019/.

Antos, Joseph. 2013. "The Medicaid Expansion Is Not Such a Good Deal for States or the Poor." *Journal of Health Politics, Policy and Law* 38, no. 1: 179–86. doi.org/10.1215/03616878-1898848.

Baicker, Katherine, Sarah L. Taubman, Heidi L. Allen, Mira Bernstein, Jonathan H. Gruber, Joseph P. Newhouse, Eric C. Schneider et al. 2013. "The Oregon Experiment—Effects of Medicaid on Clinical Outcomes." *New England Journal of Medicine* 368, no. 18: 1713–22. doi.org/10.1056/NEJMsa1212321.

Blavin, Fredric. 2016. "Association between the 2014 Medicaid Expansion and US Hospital Finances." *JAMA* 316, no. 14: 1475–83. doi.org/10.1001/jama.2016.14765.

Blavin, Fredric, Adele Shartzer, Sharon K. Long, and John Holahan. 2015. "An Early Look at Changes in Employer-Sponsored Insurance under the Affordable Care Act." *Health Affairs* 34, no. 1: 170–77. doi.org/10.1377/hlthaff.2014.1298.

Blumberg, Linda J., Matthew Buettgens, Judith Feder, and John Holahan. 2012. "Why Employers Will Continue to Provide Health Insurance: The Impact of the Affordable Care Act." *Inquiry: The Journal of Health Care Organization, Provision, and Financing* 49, no. 2: 116–16. doi.org/10.5034/inquiryjrnl_49.02.05.

Carey, Colleen M., Sarah Miller, and Laura R. Wherry. 2018. "The Impact of Insurance Expansions on the Already Insured: The Affordable Care Act and Medicare." Working Paper No. 25153, National Bureau of Economic Research. doi.org/10.3386/w25153.

Carroll, Aaron, and Austin Frakt. 2017. "Medicaid Worsens Your Health? That's a Classic Misinterpretation of Research." *New York Times*, July 3. www.nytimes.com/2017/07/03/upshot/medicaid-worsens-your-health-thats-a-classic-misinterpretation-of-research.html.

Caswell, Kyle J., and Timothy A. Waidmann. 2019. "The Affordable Care Act Medicaid Expansions and Personal Finance." *Medical Care Research and Review* 76, no. 5: 538–71. doi.org/10.1177/1077558717725164.

CBO (Congressional Budget Office). 2014a. "Insurance Coverage Provisions of the Affordable Care Act—CBO's February 2014 Baseline." www.cbo.gov/sites/default/files/recurringdata/51298-2014-02-aca.pdf (accessed February 10, 2020).

CBO (Congressional Budget Office). 2014b. "Labor Market Effects of the Affordable Care Act: Updated Estimates." February. www.cbo.gov/sites/default/files/cbofiles /attachments/45010-breakout-AppendixC.pdf.

CBO (Congressional Budget Office). 2017. "The Budget and Economic Outlook: 2017 to 2027." January 24. www.cbo.gov/publication/52370.

Cole, Megan B., Omar Galárraga, Ira B. Wilson, Brad Wright, and Amal N. Trivedi. 2017. "At Federally Funded Health Centers, Medicaid Expansion Was Associated with Improved Quality of Care." *Health Affairs* 36, no. 1. doi.org/10.1377/hlthaff .2016.0804.

Conover, Chris. 2014. "Obamacare Will Cost 2.9 Million or More Jobs a Year." *Forbes*, February 24. www.forbes.com/sites/chrisconover/2014/02/24/obamacare -will-cost-2-9-million-or-more-jobs-a-year/#238d90a059b3.

Courtemanche, Charles, James Marton, Benjamin Ukert, Aaron Yelowitz, and Daniela Zapata. 2018. "Early Effects of the Affordable Care Act on Health Care Access, Risky Health Behaviors, and Self-Assessed Health." *Southern Economic Journal* 84, no. 3: 660–61. doi.org/10.1002/soej.12245.

Cucko, Kavan, Kevin Rinz, and Benjamin Solow. 2017. "Labor Market Effects of the Affordable Care Act." US Census Bureau, July 13. www.census.gov/library /working-papers/2017/adrm/carra-wp-2017-07.html.

Cutler, David M., and Nikhil R. Sahni. 2013. "If Slow Rate of Health Care Spending Growth Persists, Projections May Be Off by $770 Billion." *Health Affairs* 32, no. 5. doi.org/10.1377/hlthaff.2012.0289.

Daw, Jamie R., and Benjamin D. Sommers. 2019. "The Affordable Care Act and Access to Care for Reproductive-aged and Pregnant Women in the United States, 2010–2016." *American Journal of Public Health* 109, no. 4: 565–71.

Duggan, Mark, Gopi S. Goda, and Emilie Jackson. 2019. "The Effects of the Affordable Care Act on Health Insurance Coverage and Labor Market Outcomes." *National Tax Journal* 72, no. 2: 261–322. doi.org/10.17310/ntj.2019.2.01.

Elmendorf, Douglas. 2011. "CBO's Analysis of the Major Health Care Legislation Enacted in March 2010." Congressional Budget Office, March 30. www.cbo.gov /sites/default/files/03-30-healthcarelegislation.pdf.

Emanuel, Ezekiel J. 2016. "How Well Is the Affordable Care Act Doing? Reasons for Optimism." *JAMA* 315, no. 13: 1331–32. doi.org/10.1001/jama.2016.2556.

Foster, Richard S. 2010. "Estimated Financial Effects of the 'Patient Protection and Affordable Care Act,' as Amended." Centers for Medicare and Medicaid Services, April 22. www.cms.gov/Research-Statistics-Data-and-Systems/Research/Actuarial Studies/downloads/PPACA_2010-04-22.pdf.

Frean, Molly, Jonathan Gruber, and Benjamin D. Sommers. 2017. "Premium Subsidies, the Mandate, and Medicaid Expansion: Coverage Effects of the Affordable Care Act." *Journal of Health Economics* 53: 72–86. doi.org/10.1016/j.jhealeco .2017.02.004.

Gara, Tom. 2013. "Union Letter: Obamacare Will 'Destroy the Very Health and Wellbeing' of Workers." *Wall Street Journal*, July 12. blogs.wsj.com/corporate -intelligence/2013/07/12/union-letter-obamacare-will-destroy-the-very-health-and -wellbeing-of-workers/.

Garrett, A. Bowen, Robert Kaestner, and Anuj Gangopadhyaya. 2017. "Recent Evidence on the ACA and Employment: Has the ACA Been a Job Killer? 2016 Update." Urban Institute, February 15. www.urban.org/research/publication/recent-evidence-aca-and-employment-has-aca-been-job-killer-2016-update.

Garthwaite, Craig, John A. Graves, Tal Gross, Zeynal Karaca, Victoria R. Marone, and Matthew J. Notowidigdo. 2019. "All Medicaid Expansions Are Not Created Equal: The Geography and Targeting of the Affordable Care Act." Working Paper No. 26289, National Bureau of Economic Research. doi.org/10.3386/w26289.

Goldin, Jacob, Ithai Z. Lurie, and Janet McCubbin. 2019. "Health Insurance and Mortality: Experimental Evidence from Taxpayer Outreach." NBER Working Paper No. 26533, National Bureau of Economic Research. www.nber.org/papers/w26533.

Gordon, Sarah H., Benjamin D. Sommers, Ira B. Wilson, and Amal N. Trivedi. 2020. "Effects Of Medicaid Expansion on Postpartum Coverage And Outpatient Utilization." *Health Affairs* 39, no. 1: 77–84.

Gottlieb, Scott. 2011. "Medicaid Is Worse than No Coverage at All." *Wall Street Journal*, March 10. www.wsj.com/articles/SB10001424052748704758904576188280858303612.

Gruber, Jonathan, and Benjamin D. Sommers. 2019. "The Affordable Care Act's Effects on Patients, Providers, and the Economy: What We've Learned So Far." *Journal of Policy Analysis and Management* 38, no. 4: 1028–52. doi.org/10.1002/pam.22158.

Gunja, Munira Z., Sara R. Collins, Michelle M. Doty, and Sophie Beutel. 2016. "Americans' Experiences with ACA Marketplace Coverage: Affordability and Provider Network Satisfaction." Commonwealth Fund, July 7. www.commonwealthfund.org/publications/issue-briefs/2016/jul/americans-experiences-aca-marketplace-coverage-affordability-and.

Holahan, John, Linda J. Blumberg, and Erik Wengle. 2017. "Premium Tax Credits Tied to Age versus Income and Available Premiums: Differences by Age, Income, and Geography." Urban Institute, May 17. www.urban.org/research/publication/premium-tax-credits-tied-age-versus-income-and-available-premiums-differences-age-income-and-geography.

Holahan, John, Erik Wengle, and Caroline Elmendorf. 2020. "Marketplace Premiums and Insurer Participation: 2017–2020." Urban Institute, January 15. www.urban.org/research/publication/marketplace-premiums-and-insurer-participation-2017-2020.

Holtz-Eakin, Douglas, and Cameron Smith. 2010. "Labor Markets and Health Care Reform: New Results." American Action Forum, May 27. americanactionforum.aaf.rededge.com/uploads/files/research/OHC_LabMktsHCR.pdf.

Hu, Luojia, Robert Kaestner, Bhashkar Mazumder, Sarah Miller, and Ashley Wong. 2018. "The Effect of the Affordable Care Act Medicaid Expansions on Financial Well-Being." *Journal of Public Economics* 163: 99–112.

Johnston, Emily M., Andrea E. Strahan, Peter Joski, Anne L. Dunlop, and E. Kathleen Adams. 2018. "Impacts of the Affordable Care Act's Medicaid Expansion on Women of Reproductive Age: Differences by Parental Status and State Policies." *Women's Health Issues* 28, no. 2: 122–29.

Kaestner, Robert A., Bowen Garrett, Jie Chen, Anuj Gangopadhyaya, and Caitlyn Fleming. 2017. "Effects of ACA Medicaid Expansions on Health Insurance Coverage and Labor Supply." *Journal of Policy Analysis and Management* 36, no. 3: 608–62. doi.org/10.1002/pam.21993.

Kaiser Family Foundation. 2013. "Summary of the Affordable Care Act." Focus on Health Reform, April 23. files.kff.org/attachment/fact-sheet-summary-of-the -affordable-care-act.

Kaiser Family Foundation. 2020. "Status of State Action on the Medicaid Expansion Decision." State Health Facts, February 7. www.kff.org/health-reform/state-indicator /state-activity-around-expanding-medicaid-under-the-affordable-care-act/.

Kessler, Glenn. 2012. "Sarah Palin, 'Death Panels,' and 'Obamacare.'" *Washington Post*, June 27. www.washingtonpost.com/blogs/fact-checker/post/sarah-palin-death -panels-and-obamacare/2012/06/27/gJQAysUP7V_blog.html.

Kirby, James B., and Jessica P. Vistnes. 2016. "Access to Care Improved for People Who Gained Medicaid or Marketplace Coverage in 2014." *Health Affairs* 35, no. 10. doi.org/10.1377/hlthaff.2016.0716.

Levy, Helen, Thomas C. Buchmueller, and Sayeh Nikpay. 2018. "Health Reform and Retirement." *Journals of Gerontology. Series B, Psychological Sciences and Social Sciences* 73, no. 4: 713–72. doi.org/10.1093/geronb/gbw115.

Loehrer, Andrew P., David C. Chang, John W. Scott, Matthew M. Hutter, Virendra I. Patel, Jeffrey E. Lee, and Benjamin D. Sommers. 2018. "Association of the Affordable Care Act Medicaid Expansion with Access to and Quality of Care for Surgical Conditions." *JAMA Surgery* 153, no. 3: e175568. doi.org/10.1001/jama-surg.2017.5568.

McMorrow, Stacey. 2010. "Will the Patient Protection and Affordable Care Act of 2010 Improve Health Outcomes for Individuals and Families?" Urban Institute, July 6. www.urban.org/research/publication/will-patient-protection-and-affordable -care-act-2010-improve-health-outcomes-individuals-and-families.

McMorrow, Stacey, and John Holahan. 2016. "The Widespread Slowdown in Health Spending Growth: Implications for Future Spending Projections and the Cost of the Affordable Care Act: An Update." Urban Institute, June 19. www.urban.org/research /publication/widespread-slowdown-health-spending-growth-implications-future -spending-projections-and-cost-affordable-care-act-update.

McMorrow, Stacey, and Daniel Polsky. 2016. "Insurance Coverage and Access to Care under the Affordable Care Act." *Issue Briefs* 21, no. 2. repository.upenn.edu /ldi_issuebriefs/2.

McMorrow, Stacey, Genevieve M. Kenney, Sharon K. Long, and Jason A. Gates. 2016. "Marketplaces Helped Drive Coverage Gains in 2015; Affordability Problems Remained." *Health Affairs* 35, no. 10: 1810–15. doi.org/10.1377/hlthaff.2016 .0941.

McMorrow, Stacey, Jason A. Gates, Sharon K. Long, and Genevieve M. Kenney. 2017. "Medicaid Expansion Increased Coverage, Improved Affordability, and Reduced Psychological Distress for Low-Income Parents." *Health Affairs* 36, no. 5: 808–88. doi.org/10.1377/hlthaff.2016.1650.

Miller, Sarah, and Laura R. Wherry. 2017. "Health and Access to Care during the First Two Years of the ACA Medicaid Expansions." *New England Journal of Medicine* 376, no. 10: 947–96. doi.org/10.1056/NEJMsa1612890.

Miller, Sarah, and Laura R. Wherry. 2019. "Four Years Later: Insurance Coverage and Access to Care Continue to Diverge between ACA Medicaid Expansion and Non-expansion States." *AEA Papers and Proceedings* 109: 327–33. doi.org/10.1257/pandp.20191046.

Miller, Sarah, Sean Altekruse, Norman Johnson, and Laura R. Wherry. 2019. "Medicaid and Mortality: New Evidence from Linked Survey and Administrative Data." Working Paper No. 26081, National Bureau of Economic Research. doi.org/10.3386/w26081.

Moriya, Asako S., Thomas M. Selden, and Kosali I. Simon. 2016. "Little Change Seen in Part-Time Employment as a Result of the Affordable Care Act." *Health Affairs* 35, no. 1: 119–13. doi.org/10.1377/hlthaff.2015.0949.

NCHS (National Center for Health Statistics). 2019. "National Health Interview Survey: Long-Term Trends in Health Insurance Coverage, 1968–2018." July. www.cdc.gov/nchs/data/nhis/health_insurance/TrendHealthInsurance1968_2018.pdf.

Nikpay, Sayeh, Seth Freedman, Helen Levy, and Thomas Buchmueller. 2017. "Effect of the Affordable Care Act Medicaid Expansion on Emergency Department Visits: Evidence from State-Level Emergency Department Databases." *Annals of Emergency Medicine* 70, no. 2: 215–25. doi.org/10.1016/j.annemergmed.2017.03.023.

Pipes, Sally. 2013. "Thanks to Obamacare, a 20,000 Doctor Shortage Is Set to Quintuple." *Forbes*, July 10. www.forbes.com/sites/sallypipes/2013/06/10/thanks-to-obamacare-a-20000-doctor-shortage-is-set-to-quintuple/#105ff46b322e.

Polsky, Daniel, Molly Candon, Brendan Saloner, Douglas Wissoker, Katherine Hempstead, Genevieve M. Kenney, and Karin Rhodes. 2017. "Changes in Primary Care Access between 2012 and 2016 for New Patients with Medicaid and Private Coverage." *JAMA Internal Medicine* 177, no. 4: 588–50. doi.org/10.1001/jama internmed.2016.9662.

Russell, Louise. 2010. *Is Prevention Better than Cure?* Washington, DC: Brookings Institution.

Selden, Thomas M., Brandy J. Lipton, and Sandra L. Decker. 2017. "Medicaid Expansion and Marketplace Eligibility Both Increased Coverage, with Trade-offs in Access, Affordability." *Health Affairs* 36, no. 12: 2069–77. doi.org/10.1377/hlthaff.2017.0830.

Shartzer, Adele, Fredric Blavin, and John Holahan. 2018. "Employer-Sponsored Insurance Stable for Low-Income Workers in Medicaid Expansion States." *Health Affairs* 37, no. 4: 607–62. doi.org/10.1377/hlthaff.2017.1205.

Simon, Kosali, Aparna Soni, and John Cawley. 2017. "The Impact of Health Insurance on Preventive Care and Health Behaviors: Evidence from the First Two Years of the ACA Medicaid Expansions." *Journal of Policy Analysis and Management* 36, no. 2: 390–47. doi.org/10.1002/pam.21972.

Sommers, Benjamin D., Munira Z. Gunja, Kenneth Finegold, and Thomas Musco. 2015. "Changes in Self-Reported Insurance Coverage, Access to Care, and Health under the Affordable Care Act." *JAMA* 314, no. 4: 366–34. doi.org/10.1001/jama.2015.8421.

Taubman, Sarah L., Heidi L. Allen, Bill J. Wright, Katherine Baicker, and Amy N. Finkelstein. 2014. "Medicaid Increases Emergency Department Use: Evidence from Oregon's Health Insurance Experiment." *Science* 343, no. 6168: 263–28. doi.org/10.1126/science.1246183.

Wehby, George L., and Wei Lyu. 2018. "The Impact of the ACA Medicaid Expansions on Health Insurance Coverage through 2015 and Coverage Disparities by Age, Race/Ethnicity, and Gender." *Health Services Research* 53, no. 2: 1248–71. doi.org/10.1111/1475-6773.12711.

Winfree, Paul. 2011. "Obamacare Tax Subsidies: Bigger Deficit, Fewer Taxpayers, Damaged Economy." Heritage Foundation, May 24. www.heritage.org/health-care-reform/report/obamacare-tax-subsidies-bigger-deficit-fewer-taxpayers-damaged-economy.

Yue, Dahai, Petra W. Rasmussen, and Ninez A. Ponce. 2018. "Racial/Ethnic Differential Effects of Medicaid Expansion on Health Care Access." *Health Services Research* 53, no. 5: 3640–56. doi.org/10.1111/1475-6773.12834.

Zewde, Naomi, Erica Eliason, Heidi Allen, and Tal Gross. 2019. "The Effects of the ACA Medicaid Expansion on Nationwide Home Evictions and Eviction Court Initiations: United States 2000–2016." *American Journal of Public Health* 109, no. 10: 1379–83. doi.org/10.2105/AJPH.2019.305230.

ACA Litigation: Politics Pursued through Other Means

Timothy Stoltzfus Jost
Washington and Lee University

Katie Keith
Georgetown University

Abstract   Despite its passage a decade ago, the Affordable Care Act (ACA) remains a politically divisive law. These political divisions have long been on display in Congress, in the White House, and in states. A long-standing stalemate in Congress—where Republicans cannot repeal the law and Democrats cannot improve it—has emboldened efforts by the executive branch to act unilaterally to implement, or undermine, the ACA. In turn, the law's opponents and supporters have turned to the courts to promote their favored policy agendas through both broadside attacks on the law and targeted challenges to its implementation. Litigation has become politics pursued through other means. These challenges have often been brought, or opposed, by state attorneys general and governors, with red-state coalitions facing off against blue-state coalitions. ACA litigation has also been characterized by forum shopping, nationwide injunctions, and questions about the court as a truly adversarial forum. This article briefly reviews the history of ACA litigation, discusses these legal norms in the context of the historic health reform law, and considers the implications of this history and the changing judiciary for future health reform efforts.

Keywords   Affordable Care Act, litigation, health reform, executive authority

The Political Context

Congress passed the Affordable Care Act (ACA) in 2010 without a single Republican vote. Although Democrats tried repeatedly to garner bipartisan support for the bill, the ACA was ultimately passed by the Democratic majorities in both chambers of Congress (McDonough 2011). During deliberations over the ACA, Democrats (joined by two independents) had a filibuster-proof majority in the US Senate and a significant majority in the

Journal of Health Politics, Policy and Law, Vol. 45, No. 4, August 2020
DOI 10.1215/03616878-8255433   © 2020 by Duke University Press

US House of Representatives. Following a loss in a special election in early 2010, Democrats in the Senate lost their 60-vote majority, ultimately forcing the use of the budget reconciliation process to pass the final ACA. This unusual process of passing the ACA has had implications for legal challenges.

Backlash, which had already been fierce throughout the health reform debate, was swift and severe. In the lead-up to the 2010 midterm elections, Democratic members of Congress faced an onslaught of criticism, and ideological opposition to the ACA helped the Tea Party movement burgeon. Months after the ACA was enacted, the Democrats lost their majority in the House and nearly lost their majority in the Senate. One study found that 25 House Democrats lost their seats due entirely to their vote on the ACA (Nyhan et al. 2012).

Those were not the only losses. Democrats also lost governor's mansions and state houses across the country. Following the 2010 election, Democrats held fewer elected offices nationwide than at any time since the 1920s (Liasson 2016). These losses had an enduring impact because Republican state legislatures and governors redrew congressional and state legislative district boundaries following the 2010 decennial census. Thus, Democrats' losses in 2010, in part due to passage of the ACA, had a decade-long impact on the political control of many states across the country and the House. Democrats would not recapture control of the House until the 2018 elections.

In 2016, President Donald Trump was elected and the Democrats lost their majority in the Senate. This left Republicans in control of both chambers of Congress and the White House from 2017 through 2019. While Republicans had repeatedly voted for legislation repealing all or part of the ACA after 2010, Republican control of both houses of Congress and the White House in 2017 was considered the party's best chance to fulfill their long-standing pledge to "repeal and replace" the ACA.

Throughout 2017, Republicans attempted, but ultimately failed, to repeal major parts of the ACA. Congress could only muster the votes to zero out the ACA's individual responsibility penalty through the Tax Cuts and Jobs Act in late 2017 (Pub. L. No. 115-97, § 11081, 131 Stat. 2054). Republicans did not take up major efforts to repeal the ACA during 2018, and Democrats retook the majority of the House in 2019 as health care became a key issue on congressional midterm races.

Where has that left the ACA itself? Other than zeroing out the individual mandate penalty in 2017, Congress has made relatively minor changes to the ACA, and the vast majority of the original law remains in place. Congress has repealed some components, such as the CLASS Act and the

Independent Payment Advisory Board. Congress has also eliminated some of the ACA's taxes, such as the health insurance tax, the medical device tax, and the Cadillac tax.

Beyond these changes, Congress has simply remained at a stalemate, where the Republicans cannot repeal the law and Democrats lack the votes necessary to improve the ACA or even to fix the law's drafting glitches. Even changes with bipartisan support have largely been viewed as non-starters, and Congress has not been able to appropriate funds to implement the ACA after the initial $1 billion of implementation funds included in the original bill.

In the face of this stalemate, the power to implement, or undermine, the ACA shifted to the executive branch and increasingly to the courts. ACA opponents have brought numerous legal challenges to the ACA and its implementing regulations, including multiple high-profile cases before the Supreme Court. Perhaps frustrated by the lack of action in Congress, the Obama and Trump administrations both attempted to maximize their executive authority under the ACA. As both administrations tested the boundaries of their authority, ACA opponents and supporters turned to the courts to promote their favored policy agendas. Litigation has become an extension of politics pursued through other means.

A Long History of ACA Litigation

Having failed to stymie the passage of the ACA in Congress, Republican-led states and ACA opponents turned immediately to the courts, asking that the ACA be struck down. Lawsuits were filed within minutes of the law's passage, claiming that the ACA or various provisions of the ACA were unconstitutional, and they continue to this day.

Obama-Era Litigation

The first challenge to reach the Supreme Court, *National Federation of Independent Business v. Sebelius (NFIB)* (567 US 519 [2012]), was led by the attorney general of Florida joined by 25 other Republican attorneys general, the National Federation of Independent Businesses, and individual plaintiffs. In *NFIB*, the Supreme Court held that Congress lacked the authority to adopt the individual mandate under its interstate commerce authority but that Congress had validly exercised its power to tax individuals who failed to have coverage.

The Supreme Court further held that Congress did not have the authority to require states to participate in the ACA's Medicaid expansion, opening up another pathway for Republican-led states to resist the ACA by refusing to expand Medicaid. While Democratic-led states quickly expanded Medicaid, many Republican-led states balked. Even today, 14 states have yet to expand their Medicaid programs, and voters in an additional state (Nebraska) passed a referendum requiring Medicaid expansion that the state has yet to implement (Kaiser Family Foundation 2020).

The litigation did not stop there. Two other ACA-related challenges have been heard by the Supreme Court: *Burwell v. Hobby Lobby Stores, Inc.* (134 S. Ct. 2751 [2014]) and *King v. Burwell* (135 S. Ct. 2480 [2015]). In both cases, the plaintiffs did not directly attack the constitutionality of the ACA or one of its provisions but, rather, challenged the scope of a regulation adopted to implement the ACA. Both cases were brought by private parties rather than state attorneys general and were motivated by ideological opposition to the ACA. Relevant to *King*, for instance, libertarian advocates told red states they could effectively opt out of the ACA by refusing to establish their own marketplace (Cannon 2013).

In *Hobby Lobby*, for-profit companies challenged the applicability to them of the ACA's preventive services coverage regulations requiring employer and university health plans to cover contraceptives for their employees and students.[1] The Supreme Court held that a regulatory accommodation adopted by the Obama administration for certain types of religious employers should extend to closely held for-profit corporations that object to contraceptive coverage for religious reasons. As discussed more below, lawsuits over the scope of the contraceptive mandate have continued; this issue was considered again by the Supreme Court in *Zubik v. Burwell* in 2016 (136 S. Ct. 1557) and will be before the Court once more during its 2019–20 term when it considers *Little Sisters of the Poor v. Pennsylvania* (No. 19-431).

In *King*, the plaintiffs challenged an Internal Revenue Service regulation that authorized the availability of premium tax credits in all states, regardless of whether the state opted for a state- or federally run Health Insurance Marketplace. The plaintiffs asserted that these subsidies were available only in states with a state-run marketplace. Had they won, most states and millions of people would have been left without access to

---

1. Approximately 100 lawsuits were filed, about half by for-profit companies arguing that they should be granted an exception to the requirement and the other half by religious organizations protesting the notice requirements to claim an exception for nonprofits.

subsidies. Chief Justice Roberts ultimately held that the federal market-place could offer premium tax credits, bringing an end to the litigation.

At the end of his opinion in *King*, the Chief Justice noted that "in a democracy, the power to make the law rests with those chosen by the people. . . . We must respect the role of the Legislature, and take care not to undo what it has done. . . . Congress passed the Affordable Care Act to improve health insurance markets, not to destroy them" (135 S. Ct. at 2496). This message was largely perceived as a warning to would-be challengers that the Supreme Court had no interest in striking down the ACA.

This warning has not been heeded. Litigation continued, although lawsuits generally focused more on Obama-administration interpretations in implementing regulations and guidance than on constitutional challenges. Legal challenges have addressed a wide range of issues, including the risk corridors program, the risk adjustment program, whether the administration could make cost-sharing reduction payments to insurers, nondiscrimination protections, and the decision to allow the continuation of non-ACA-compliant "grandmothered" health insurance plans.[2] These lawsuits have had mixed results, and while none has proven fatal to the ACA, they have led to uncertainty for insurers, regulators, and consumers alike. These challenges have also contributed to a sense that the ACA is not a legitimate law and have undermined public confidence in the ACA.

One of these lawsuits, seeking unpaid risk corridor payments, will be decided by the Supreme Court in 2020. The temporary risk corridors program was designed to help stabilize the ACA Marketplace, and insurers participated in the Marketplace in part due to the expectation that full risk corridor payments would be made. The Centers for Medicare and Medicaid Services (CMS) later decided not to pay out more than what was received from insurers, while Congress passed a series of appropriation riders that prevented CMS from paying out more than it collected. Given high losses in the early years of the Marketplace, insurers were owed more than $12 billion in unpaid risk corridor payments. They sued, resulting in mixed results at the court of claims level and a loss at the federal circuit in a 2–1 decision (Moda Health Plan v. United States, 892 F.3d 1311 [Fed. Cir. 2018]). The Supreme Court agreed to review this decision, and a ruling is

---

2. "Grandmothered" plans are health plans that were issued after the ACA was enacted in 2010 but before the law's major reforms went into effect in 2014. These plans thus have to comply with some, but not all, of the ACA's most significant consumer protections, and they would have been made illegal in 2014 but were allowed to continue by administrative guidance. They are distinguished from "grandfathered" plans, which existed on the day the ACA was enacted and were allowed to continue under certain circumstances.

expected in 2020. The Supreme Court's decision could have significant implications that extend beyond the realm of the ACA and impact the future of public-private partnerships.

Trump-Era Litigation

The 2016 election ushered in a new era in ACA litigation. Beginning in 2017, the Trump administration acted to exploit or create ACA loopholes. President Trump issued executive orders directing federal regulators to undermine the ACA (Exec. Order No. 13765, 82 Fed. Reg. 8351 [Jan. 24, 2017]; Exec. Order No. 13813, 82 Fed. Reg. 48385 [Oct. 17, 2017]). In response to these executive orders and other directives from the White House, federal agencies rescinded Obama-era ACA interpretations while broadening or creating new exemptions to the ACA's consumer protections.

In response to an executive order, federal agencies issued new rules to dramatically expand the availability of short-term limited-duration health insurance and association health plans (Short-Term, Limited Duration Insurance, 83 Fed. Reg. 38212 [Aug. 3, 2018]; Definition of "Employer" under Section 3[5] of ERISA-Association Health Plans, 83 Fed. Reg. 28912 [June 21, 2018]). These plans are not part of the individual or small-group market single-risk pool and do not have to comply with all of the ACA's most significant consumer protections, making them attractive to younger, healthier people in search of lower premiums. This risk of adverse selection results in higher premiums for individuals with preexisting medical conditions and thus bigger federal outlays through higher Marketplace subsidies.

Both of these new rules have been challenged in court, with mixed results. Democratic attorneys general challenged the new rule on association health plans, arguing that the rule was inconsistent with the text and purpose of the Employee Retirement Income Security Act of 1974 and the ACA. The district court agreed, setting aside major portions of the Trump administration's rule (New York v. Department of Labor, 363 F. Supp. 3d 109 [D.D.C. 2019]). The new rule on short-term limited-duration health insurance was challenged by a coalition of safety-net health plans and patient advocates who asserted that the rule creates a loophole to the ACA that hurts patients with preexisting conditions. The district court disagreed, upholding the rule as a valid interpretation of federal law (Association for Community Affiliated Plans v. Department of Treasury, 392 F. Supp. 3d 22 [D.D.C. 2019]). Both decisions were appealed to the Court of Appeals for the D.C. Circuit.

The Trump administration has also encouraged states to consider new initiatives that seem to run afoul of federal law. Federal regulators have encouraged states to apply for state innovation waivers that may not comply with statutory requirements under section 1332 of the ACA, including requirements that state waiver programs provide coverage that is at least as comprehensive and affordable as ACA coverage and cover at least a comparable number of people. To date, only Georgia has sought such a broader waiver under the ACA, which CMS has not yet approved. CMS has approved novel waivers in the Medicaid context, allowing states to impose work requirements on Medicaid recipients. These waivers have so far been successfully challenged in court as inconsistent with the purpose of the Medicaid Act and thus unauthorized under federal law.

A separate lawsuit, known as the "Take Care" case, challenges a suite of changes made by the Trump administration to undermine the ACA. The plaintiffs—five cities and two individuals—challenge the administration's decision to stop making cost-sharing reduction payments to insurers, budget cuts for Marketplace advertising and in-person enrollment, a shortened open enrollment period, and the Department of Justice's refusal to defend the ACA in court. They argue that these changes, among others, violate the Constitution's requirement that the president "take care that the laws be faithfully executed" (U.S. Const. art. II, § 3) and that the administration is attempting to nullify the ACA through executive action.

Other Trump-era ACA lawsuits include challenges to new rules that would dramatically expand exemptions to the contraceptive mandate and the administration's decision to cease making cost-sharing reduction payments to insurers. Other non-ACA Trump administration health policy priorities—ranging from rules governing provider conscience protections to drug pricing transparency—have also been challenged in court.

In the meantime, all eyes are on *Texas v. United States*, a third global challenge to the ACA. In the Tax Cuts and Jobs Act, Congress—after multiple high-profile failed attempts to "repeal and replace" the ACA— set the penalty for failing to have health insurance at $0. Twenty Republican attorneys general and governors, later joined by two individuals in Texas, argue that the penaltyless mandate can no longer be upheld as a tax under *NFIB*. Because the mandate cannot be sustained as a tax, they argue that it is unconstitutional and should be struck down. They further argue that the mandate is so essential to the rest of the ACA that the entire law should be invalidated. As discussed more below, the district court agreed with the plaintiffs (Texas v. United States, 340 F. Supp. 3d 579 [N.D. Tex. 2018]) and the case was appealed to the Fifth Circuit. In December of

2019, the Fifth Circuit partially upheld the district court's decision that the mandate is now unconstitutional but remanded the case to the district court to reconsider how much of the rest of the ACA should also be invalidated (Texas v. United States, No. 19-10011, 2019 WL 6888446 [5th Cir. Dec. 18, 2019]). A coalition of states—led by the attorney general of California—and the House of Representatives appealed the Fifth Circuit's decision to the Supreme Court, which agreed to hear the appeal during its next term.

Legal Norms and the Role of the Judiciary

Courts have long been used as a means to promote preferred policy agendas. Thus, some tools used in ACA litigation, ranging from coalitions of state attorneys general to forum shopping, are by no means unique to the ACA. Litigation using these tools has been particularly apparent in other areas of law that raise important and divisive public policy issues, such as immigration or environmental law, and ACA litigation to some extent relies on precedents from these other areas of law. However, a long and sustained history of ACA litigation offers a unique case study in the political use of the courts, modern legal norms, and the role of the judiciary in resolving politically motivated challenges and mediating policy disagreements. This section discusses some of the hallmarks of ACA litigation in the context of ACA litigation writ large and the latest global challenge to the law, *Texas v. United States*.

Coalitions of Attorneys General

Challenges to the ACA and its implementation are regularly brought by state attorneys general: Republican during the Obama administration and Democratic during the Trump administration. State attorneys general also file amicus briefs in support of or in opposition to litigation and intervene as defendants where the Trump administration refuses to defend the law. Although some cases have been pursued by single state attorneys general, most have involved coalitions of states.

Further underscoring the political undertone of these challenges, some coalitions include governors of states where the attorney general is of a different party, and some attorneys general have left or joined coalitions following an election and change in party affiliation. The prominent role of states in bringing these lawsuits has led to questions about whether states, as employers or on the basis of other claimed injury, have standing to bring such challenges in the first place.

Coalitions of state attorneys general have played a particularly important role in some of the major ACA challenges that have come before the Supreme Court. The *NFIB* challenge was initially brought by 26 Republican attorneys general and defended in an amicus brief before the Supreme Court by 12 Democratic attorneys general and a governor (Brief for California and 12 Other States Supporting Respondents). *Texas* was initially brought by 20 Republican attorneys general and governors. Even before the Trump administration declined to defend major parts of the ACA, a coalition of 17 Democratic attorneys general, led by California, asked to intervene in *Texas*. Following the 2018 midterm elections, two Republican states withdrew as plaintiffs and four additional Democratic attorneys general asked to intervene, resulting in 18 Republican-represented states challenging the ACA and 21 Democratic-represented states defending the ACA.

Republican attorneys general in Texas and Wisconsin have been particularly active in challenging the ACA and Obama-era interpretations of the law. The attorney general of Texas has challenged the individual mandate, nondiscrimination regulations, and the health insurance tax. On the other end of the spectrum, Democratic attorneys general in California and New York have led coalitions to defend the ACA and challenged Trump-era efforts to undermine the law. These attorneys general have challenged recent rules to expand access to association health plans, exemptions to the contraceptive mandate, and a new provider conscience rule.

Even where state attorneys general are not directly involved in a lawsuit, many file amicus briefs in support of the plaintiffs or federal government. In *Hobby Lobby*, amicus briefs were filed by 21 Republican attorneys general in favor of the plaintiffs and 16 Democratic attorneys general in support of the government (Brief for Michigan, Ohio, and 18 Other States Supporting Respondents; Brief for Oklahoma Supporting Respondents; Brief for California and 15 Other States Supporting Petitioners). A similar pattern emerged in *King*, which was brought by private parties (not states), although two similar cases were filed by the attorneys general of Oklahoma and Indiana as state employers (Oklahoma ex rel. Pruitt v. Burwell, 51 F. Supp. 3d 1080 [E.D. Okla. 2014]; Indiana v. Internal Revenue Service, 38 F. Supp. 3d 1003 [S.D. Ind. 2014]). Before the Supreme Court, 6 Republican attorneys general filed an amicus brief in support of the plaintiffs compared to 23 Democratic attorneys general in support of the government (Brief for Oklahoma and 5 Other States Supporting Petitioners; Brief for the Commonwealth of Virginia and 22 Other States Supporting Respondents).

Forum Shopping

ACA challenges have also been characterized by forum shopping, where a plaintiff files a lawsuit in a certain jurisdiction where a judge is likely to issue a favorable ruling. This strategy has been used effectively by both supporters and opponents of the ACA.

Forum shopping has gone hand in hand with challenges brought by attorneys general. The Texas attorney general consistently files lawsuits in the northern district of Texas, resulting in many of these challenges being heard by Judge Reed O'Connor, who has uniformly found the ACA and its implementing regulations to be invalid. For years, Judge O'Connor was the only judge in the Wichita Falls division of the northern district, meaning challenges brought by Texas there were virtually guaranteed to be heard in his courtroom. Since 2015, nearly half of all challenges to the federal government brought by the Texas attorney general—on the ACA and beyond—have been heard by Judge O'Connor (Platoff 2018).

Given this, it is unsurprising that Judge O'Connor has played a central role in *Texas*, which was filed in the northern district by the Texas attorney general. In December 2018, Judge O'Connor issued an opinion agreeing with Texas and the other plaintiffs that the penaltyless individual mandate was unconstitutional and declared the entire ACA to be invalid. In December of 2019, the Fifth Circuit upheld Judge O'Connor's ruling that the mandate was unconstitutional but sent the case back to him to reconsider how much of the rest of the ACA should be invalidated with it. As noted above, the Supreme Court has agreed to review this decision.

ACA supporters also strategically file lawsuits in jurisdictions that are perceived to be sympathetic. Challenges have been brought in courts in California, the District of Columbia, Maryland, and New York. However, there is no analogue to the northern district of Texas for ACA supporters; said another way, there is no single court or judge that has heard a significant number of ACA challenges brought by supporters of the law.

Nationwide Injunctions

ACA litigation has also resulted in a number of nationwide injunctions to halt executive branch policies. Legal scholars have hotly debated the propriety of nationwide injunctions, which have been issued with increased frequency in recent years (Bray 2017; Malveaux 2017). Concerns about the effect of nationwide injunctions led the Department of Justice to issue new litigation guidelines criticizing this form of "overbroad injunctive relief"

(Sessions 2018). Nationwide injunctions have been issued against both Obama- and Trump-era policies to implement the ACA. In other instances, courts have vacated all or parts of regulations, effectively invalidating federal rules nationwide.

Most of the nationwide injunctions issued against Obama-era policies were issued by Judge O'Connor. He enjoined parts of implementing regulations for ACA nondiscrimination protections and, more recently, the contraceptive mandate (Franciscan Alliance v. Burwell, 227 F. Supp. 3d 660 [N.D. Tex. 2016]; DeOtte v. Azar, 393 F. Supp. 3d 490 [N.D. Tex. 2019]). In *Texas*, Judge O'Connor was asked to issue a nationwide injunction but instead issued a declaratory judgment that the entire ACA was invalid. He did so in part because the Department of Justice intended to treat a declaratory judgment like a nationwide injunction (Keith 2018).

Other courts have enjoined Trump-era policies on expanded exemptions to the contraceptive mandate and vacated new rules on new association health plans. Courts in California and Pennsylvania issued nationwide injunctions against interim final rules and, later, final rules allowing employers with religious and moral objections to the contraceptive mandate to refuse compliance. On appeal, the Ninth Circuit limited the scope of the district court's nationwide injunction to only the represented plaintiff states, while the Third Circuit upheld a nationwide injunction against the rules in all 50 states (California v. Department of Health and Human Services, No. 19-15072 [9th Cir. 2019]; Pennsylvania v. Trump, 930 F.3d 543 [3rd Cir. 2019]). As noted above, the Supreme Court agreed to hear an appeal (filed by Little Sisters of the Poor and the Trump administration) of the Third Circuit's decision during the court's 2019–20 term.

Agreements between Plaintiffs and the Federal Government

An emerging issue under the Trump administration has been collusive litigation, where plaintiffs file a lawsuit against the federal government, which then agrees with the plaintiffs and refuses to defend the challenged action or regulation. This occurred in *Texas*, where the Trump administration, first in part and later in whole, agreed that the penaltyless individual mandate is unconstitutional and inseverable from the rest of the law.

In *Texas*, the Trump administration justified its decision not to defend the ACA by citing the Obama administration's decision not to defend the constitutionality of the Defense of Marriage Act. However, the Trump administration has taken collusive positions in additional, lesser known cases that have not turned on constitutional questions. In at least two additional cases—one on the contraceptive mandate and one on the ACA's nondiscrimination protections—the Trump administration has agreed with the plaintiffs that parts of Obama-era regulations should be invalidated. In those instances, the court has delayed or refused to allow outside parties to intervene in the litigation, leaving no party in the lawsuit to defend against or appeal anti-ACA decisions.

Implications for Future Health Reform Efforts

The ACA experience should inform future health reform efforts. The onslaught of litigation over the ACA, while not fatal to the law, has hindered its effectiveness and public confidence in the law and helped the ACA to remain salient as a highly partisan issue. Even 10 years after its enactment, the divide over the ACA between red states and blue states continues to be litigated in *Texas*, which remains the most significant ACA legal challenge to watch.

One irony of the ACA is that its attempt to minimize disruption and build on the current private health insurance system may have generated more legal questions and challenges than if Congress had more broadly leveraged a decidedly federal (and thus perhaps more legally sound program) like Medicare. The ACA also deferred a number of ACA implementation and design decisions to states by extending the existing cooperative federalist framework for regulating private health insurance and shared federal-state oversight of the Medicaid program. While perhaps politically expedient, this enabled dramatically different results in different states, making the ACA much more successful in states that embraced it than those that did not. This differential success rate may have contributed to ongoing legal challenges over the law.

Yet another lesson, although perhaps a dissatisfying one, is that partisan reform is very risky. The ACA, passed solely with Democratic support, remains a hyperpartisan issue even after 20 million people have gained coverage and the law has been baked into the nation's health care fabric over the past 10 years. Fervor over the ACA and the future of health care has shaped political control of state legislatures and an entire chamber of Congress, with Democrats swept out of power during the 2010 midterm elections due to anti-ACA sentiment, only to be swept back into power during the 2018 midterm elections due to opposition to Republican efforts to roll back the law's protections.

On the one hand, the past decade of legal and political battles over the ACA could underscore the need for truly bipartisan health care reforms. Congress has, for instance, still been able to achieve bipartisan agreement in other health care contexts such as the Medicare program and the Twenty-First Century Cures Act of 2016. These reforms enjoy widespread public support and have not faced the same legal or political challenges that the ACA has faced.

On the other hand, the decade of battles over the ACA could suggest that comprehensive bipartisan reform of our health care system, or even bipartisan efforts to expand further access to health coverage and care, is simply not possible now or in the foreseeable future. This recognition is animating some of the bolder proposals put forward by Democratic presidential candidates in 2020, such as Sen. Elizabeth Warren's (D-MA) explicit plans to leverage the budget reconciliation process—with its advantage of only needing a majority of votes in the Senate—to advance Medicare buy-in and public option proposals.

As with the ACA, future health reform laws, especially partisan ones, may face legal challenges. These challenges might focus on the law's fundamental statutory scheme or more broadly take issue with implementation of such a law and limits on executive authority. Many big health policy advances, especially those being discussed in the lead-up to the 2020 presidential election, such as Medicare for All, would defer a significant degree of flexibility and implementing authority to federal agencies. To the extent that private parties or states take issue with implementation of a new federal health care law, lawsuits could follow. Moreover, even if reform were to be built on an established federal program like Medicare, opponents will likely come up with novel legal theories to challenge it, and courts may reach surprising results, as the Supreme Court did in limiting Medicaid expansion in *NFIB*. Challenges over the ACA have been creative, and politically motivated legal challenges will undoubtedly continue regardless of the type of reform advanced by Congress or a new administration.

For this reason alone, reformers should not ignore the Trump administration's reshaping of the federal judiciary. President Trump continues to appoint record numbers of judges to courts across the country (Wheeler 2019). Given the degree of health policy we are doing by litigation, it seems inevitable that these new judges will consider challenges over the ACA and future health reform efforts.

■ ■ ■

Timothy Stoltzfus Jost is an emeritus professor at the Washington and Lee University School of Law. He is a coauthor of, *Health Law*, a casebook used widely throughout the United States in teaching health law, now in its eighth edition. He has written numerous monographs on legal issues in health care reform for national organizations and until 2018 blogged regularly on regulatory issues for *Health Affairs*, where he is a contributing editor. He is a member of the National Academy of Medicine and is widely quoted in the media on health reform issues.
jostt@wlu.edu

Katie Keith is an associate research professor at Georgetown University's Center on Health Insurance Reforms and teaches courses on the Affordable Care Act and LGBT health law and policy at Georgetown University Law Center. She specializes in state and federal implementation of the ACA and provides "Following the ACA" rapid response analysis for *Health Affairs*. She is an appointed consumer representative to the National Association of Insurance Commissioners and maintains an active consulting practice, where she advises nonprofits and foundations on health care issues.

References

Bray, Samuel L. 2017. "Multiple Chancellors: Reforming the National Injunction." *Harvard Law Review* 131, no. 2: 418–82.

Cannon, Michael F. 2013. *Fifty Vetoes: How States Can Stop the Obama Health Care Law*. Washington, DC: Cato Institute. www.cato.org/sites/cato.org/files/pubs/pdf/50-vetoes-white-paper_1.pdf.

Kaiser Family Foundation. 2020. *Status of State Medicaid Expansion Decisions: Interactive Map*. January 10. www.kff.org/medicaid/issue-brief/status-of-state-medicaid-expansion-decisions-interactive-map/.

Keith, Katie. 2018. "Judge Hears Oral Arguments in *Texas v. United States*." *Health Affairs Blog*, September 10. www.healthaffairs.org/do/10.1377/hblog20180910.861789/full/.

Liasson, Mara. 2016. "The Democratic Party Got Crushed during the Obama Presidency. Here's Why." National Public Radio, March 4. www.npr.org/2016/03/04/469052020/the-democratic-party-got-crushed-during-the-obama-presidency-heres-why.

Malveaux, Suzette M. 2017. "Class Actions, Civil Rights, and the National Injunction." *Harvard Law Review* 131: 56–64. harvardlawreview.org/2017/12/class-actions-civil-rights-national-injunction/.

McDonough, John E. 2011. *Inside National Health Reform*. Berkeley: University of California Press.

Nyhan, Brendan, Eric McGhee, John Sides, Seth Masket, and Steven Greene. 2012. "One Vote Out of Step? The Effects of Salient Roll Call Votes in the 2010 Election." *American Politics Research* 40, no. 5: 844–79.

Platoff, Emma. 2018. "By Gutting Obamacare, Judge Reed O'Connor Handed Texas a Win. It Wasn't the First Time." *Texas Tribune*, December 19. www.texastribune .org/2018/12/19/reed-oconnor-federal-judge-texas-obamacare-forum-shopping -ken-paxton/.

Sessions, Jeff. 2018. "Litigation Guidelines for Cases Presenting the Possibility of Nationwide Injunctions." US Justice Department, September 13. www.justice.gov /opa/press-release/file/1093881/download.

Wheeler, Russell. 2019. "Trump's Judicial Appointments Record at the August Recess: A Little Less than Meets the Eye." Brookings, August 8. www.brookings .edu/blog/fixgov/2019/08/08/trumps-judicial-appointments-record-at-the-august -recess-a-little-less-than-meets-the-eye/.

Promise, Performance, and Litigation
The ACA's Choice Problem

Allison K. Hoffman
University of Pennsylvania

Abstract   The Affordable Care Act (ACA) is in many ways a success. Millions more Americans now have access to health care, and the ACA catalyzed advances in health care delivery reform. Simultaneously, it has reinforced and bolstered a problem at the heart of American health policy and regulation: a love affair with choice. The ACA's insurance reforms doubled down on the particularly American obsession with choice. This article describes three ways in which that doubling down is problematic for the future of US health policy. First, pragmatically, health policy theory predicts that choice among health plans will produce tangible benefits that it does not actually produce. Most people do not like choosing among health plan options, and many people—even if well educated and knowledgeable—do not make good choices. Second, creating the regulatory structures to support these choices built and reinforced a massive market bureaucracy. Finally, and most important, philosophically and sociologically the ACA reinforces the idea that the goal of health regulation should be to preserve choice, even when that choice is empty. This vicious cycle seems likely to persist based on the lead up to the 2020 presidential election.

Keywords   Affordable Care Act, ACA, choice, managed competition, health insurance

The Affordable Care Act (ACA) is in many ways a success. Millions more Americans now have access to health care, and it catalyzed advances in delivery reform. Simultaneously, the ACA has reinforced and bolstered a problem at the heart of American health policy and regulation: a love affair with choice. More specifically, the problem is sanctifying the idea that choice of health insurance plans is valuable. When it comes to some aspects

Journal of Health Politics, Policy and Law, Vol. 45, No. 4, August 2020
DOI 10.1215/03616878-8255445   © 2020 by Duke University Press

of their health care, people may genuinely appreciate options and being able to make choices that leave them better off. Some people care about selecting a doctor they like and trust or who is convenient to their home or work. Many people care about reproductive choice. Most of us value the ability to decline care we don't want. But very few people value choosing a health plan, in and of itself.

The ACA's insurance reforms doubled down on the particularly American obsession with choice. This article describes three ways in which that doubling down is problematic for the future of US health policy. First, pragmatically, health policy theory predicts that choice among health plans will produce tangible benefits that it does not in fact produce. Most people do not like choosing among health plan options, and many people—even if well educated and knowledgeable—do not make good choices. Second, creating the regulatory structures to support choices has built and reinforced a massive market bureaucracy, which I describe in detail elsewhere (Hoffman 2019b). Finally, and most important, philosophically and sociologically the ACA reinforces the idea that the goal of health regulation should be to preserve choice, even when that choice is empty. This vicious cycle seems likely to persist based on the lead up to the 2020 presidential election.

The Pragmatic Problem with Choice of Health Plan

Mostly simply, the problem of choice of health plan is that it does not—and cannot—work in practice as anticipated in theory. The primary goal of the ACA was to reduce the number of uninsured and underinsured Americans through two main pathways: a Medicaid expansion and making individual (nongroup) health insurance more accessible and affordable.

The policy design that motivated the latter—the expansion of the individual market—was modeled off of a similar reform in Massachusetts in 2006 and based loosely on the theory of managed competition, most often associated with Stanford economist Alain C. Enthoven (1978a, 1978b, 1993). The oversimplified idea is that when consumers choose among health plans in a marketplace that is carefully regulated, they will make choices based on their preferences. Since most people will presumably choose plans where they get better care at lower costs, insurers will design and offer higher-value plans to compete for their business.

Enthoven (1978b: 718) initially called the idea "Consumer-Choice Health Plan" and explained, "What distinguishes [this plan] from the others is that it seeks to give the consumer a choice from among alternative systems for organizing and financing care, and to allow him to benefit from his economizing choices." For example, Enthoven (1978a: 652) stated that if people wanted a plan that prioritized better access to home health care or ambulatory care over, for example, hospitalization, they could choose it.

Enthoven's implicit assumption was that a tightly managed plan with an integrated delivery system, like a staff-model health maintenance organization, would prevail. He imagined plans where primary care providers would benefit financially if they reduced their patients' excessive use of expensive specialty and inpatient care. If this reduction lowered plan spending but not quality, people would increasingly want these plans. Enthoven (1978b: 715) sought to mobilize choice in part to correct the thorny problems of overreliance on specialists and fee-for-service medicine.

Managed competition has influenced nearly every major health financing reform effort of the past decades. It graduated to the policy main stage in the early 1990s, when it was incorporated into the blueprint for President Clinton's attempt at health reform, the Health Security Act (H.R. 3600, 103d Cong. [1993–94]). Although that reform failed, the idea lived on in the design of the Medicare Part D prescription drug coverage and Medicare Advantage, where Medicare beneficiaries can choose among plans administered by private health insurance companies.

Most recently, managed competition emerged in the ACA's health insurance exchanges, or Marketplace, where people could shop for plans. The ground rules for insurers were similar to what Enthoven (1978b: 713–14) described in his first blueprint, mandating that they accept any applicant during an open enrollment period (guaranteed issue), requiring "community-rated" premiums that do not vary based on health status, and placing limits on out-of-pocket spending. Like Enthoven's vision, the ACA was designed with the idea that consumers' choices would drive value in a managed, competitive insurance marketplace.

The problem for the ACA, and with all of the versions of managed competition prior, is that it does not work as imagined. The reasons are many. The first problem is a flawed market, where choices do not resound as clearly as Enthoven envisioned. He imagined consumers' signals to insurers would prompt insurers to transform health care financing and delivery. Although less true when Enthoven first wrote, providers have accreted substantial market power through consolidation, undermining insurers' negotiating power.[1]

---

1. Vogt and Town (2006: 1, 6) document changes in concentration during the 1990s. Gaynor and Town (2012) report that hospital consolidation increased the price of hospital care and sometimes decreases quality. Dafny (2014: 198) states that "the last hospital-merger wave (in the 1990s) led to substantial price increases with little or no countervailing benefit."

The ACA, as designed, only exacerbates this power imbalance. Managed competition relies on having multiple insurers competing for customers, but the more insurers there are in the Marketplace, the less any one of them enrolls enough subscribers to gain bargaining power. Furthermore, the ACA's exchanges reach a small slice of the population: initial best-case scenario estimates were about 24.7 million people enrolled by 2019 (CBO 2010). Actual annual enrollment to date is less than half that number (Kaiser Family Foundation 2019). With enrollees divided among 50 states, insurers gain little leverage to negotiate with behemoth hospital systems.

Even without faulty markets, the second major problem would be fatal: Enthoven's idealized consumer, who chooses smartly among plans, does not—and will never—exist (Glied 2007). This problem is multilayered. First, neoclassical economics assumes that consumers have well-ordered preferences, or "tastes," that are genuinely aligned with their interests. Yet, people do not have exogenous preferences among systems of financing and organizing care. Most people have never experienced home health care or ambulatory care versus hospitalization. It is difficult to get a sense of willingness to pay for something that is intangible.

Second, if people did have well-ordered preferences, most would struggle to translate them into plan choice. Most people do not understand the basic and defining features of health insurance plans, such as how much a plan costs and what benefits are covered (Garnick et al. 1993: 206). In a survey of insured adults, only 14% correctly answered four simple multiple-choice questions about cost-sharing features, such as a deductible, that are central to understanding the value of the plan (Loewenstein et al. 2013: 855). Yet, people overestimated their understanding, which suggests many would not seek help or education even if offered.

Third, choosing a health plan requires making calculations regarding deductibles, cost sharing, premiums, and probability that exceed many Americans' literacy and numeracy skills (Nelson et al. 2008; Peters and Levin 2008; Reyna et al. 2009: 945–46). Even college-educated Americans show surprisingly high levels of error on simple arithmetic tests (Nelson et al. 2008: 263).

Fourth, even without these fundamental problems, choosing health insurance has all of the telltale characteristics that impair rational decision making, sometimes referred to as cognitive biases. For example, people are overly optimistic about their own health (Weinstein 1980), which could prompt them to underinvest in health insurance. People also struggle to factor risk into decision making, an element central, of course, to health insurance choices.[2] This explains in part why young, healthy people may forgo buying health insurance, even when it's cheap.

Not surprisingly, a volume of empirical work documents that people, regardless of education, income, or smarts, routinely make poor choices among health plans. These poor choices persist even when options are simplified. And they persist even in the face of substantial choice architecture and simplification to improve decision making, which caused Bhargava and Loewenstein (2015: 2506) to conclude that "the main barrier to financially efficient choice was not the number of options confronting employees, nor the transparency of their presentation, but rather the . . . lack of basic understanding of health insurance."

A few representative studies, among the many dozens documenting this unyielding failure, illustrate the problem. One study simulated the purchase of an ACA plan using only participants who passed a screening test for basic insurance literacy (Johnson et al. 2013). These more-literate-than-average subjects still selected the best choice only about half of the time. Wharton business school students got it wrong over one-quarter of the time. Short of defaulting people into the right option, choice architecture tools, like just-in-time calculators and tutorials, produced little improvement.

As another example, in the University of Michigan employee plan, over one-third of enrollees selected a plan that was identical to another option in every way except that it had a more restricted provider network (Sinaiko and Hirth 2011: 453). There was no scenario in which a worker would be better off enrolled in this plan, yet a large number of employees selected it. Another study of a large US firm found that most employees chose a worse option and, as a result, paid on average 24% more than they should have on premiums (Bhargava, Loewenstein, and Sydnor 2017: 1325). Lower-income employees were more likely to make a bad choice.

Similar results occur in the Medicare market, where beneficiaries choose among private prescription drug plans. One study revealed that 73% of enrollees could have chosen a plan with lower premiums with no risk of spending more on prescription drugs during the year (Abaluck and Gruber 2011: 379). Another estimated that less than 10% of enrollees in Medicare drug plans choose their least-expensive option (Heiss et al. 2012).

---

2. Kahneman and Tversky (1979: 264) indicate that people make choices inconsistent with their own expected utility when navigating risky options.

Once Medicare beneficiaries choose plans, they usually do not switch during subsequent open enrollment periods (Koma et al. 2019), even when they would be made better off by doing so (Afendulis, Sinaiko, and Frank 2017).

People choose ACA plans that will cost them more in the long run (Avalere Health 2015; Fung et al. 2017). As many as one-third of people enroll in a plan with the lowest monthly premiums but that make them ineligible for significant cost-sharing reductions that would limit their out-of-pocket spending when they use care. Others choose health plans that are not aligned with their own stated medical needs and preferences. One simulation of an ACA exchange found that 40% of respondents chose a plan that would cost them at least $500 more than another option based on their self-reported health needs (Barnes, Hanoch, and Rice 2014: 67). In a different simulated study, only one-third of respondents chose the cost-minimizing plan, based on their own anticipated medical care need (Bhargava, Loewenstein, and Benartzi 2017). Forty-three percent of people overinsured, on average overspending by 24% or $1324 on premiums, and nearly a quarter underinsured. The authors estimated that if all people buying plans on the ACA exchanges had similar error rates as the study population, "the result would be roughly $7.1 billion of excess spending each year, borne by a population with low to moderate incomes" (10).

Thus, managed competition, in practice, is not fostering meaningful choice or making people better off.

The Bureaucratic Problem with Choice of Health Plan

These choice-venerating policies, in turn, create larger institutional problems, what I call health care's market bureaucracy (Hoffman 2019b). Markets do not exist in isolation (Vogel 2018). Regulations determine the bounds of competition (Marone 1994). Establishing these bounds for the ACA exchanges was a major lift, guided by no less than 100 pages of the ACA and Herculean regulatory efforts interpreting these pages. To set up and run the ACA exchanges, the federal government has spent tens of billions of dollars (Mach and Redhead 2014), and states have spent additional billions of dollars; California estimates annual costs of $350 million to run its exchange (Covered California 2018).

When exchanges falter or ground rules change, updates have required armies of health regulators, reams of regulation, and seemingly endless evaluation and adjustment by technocratic experts (Hoffman 2019a).

Under the Obama administration alone, the Department of Health and Human Services issued 24 new rules and 64 guidance documents on the exchanges,[3] with parallel efforts in many states. The Trump administration continues apace, undoing much of the Obama administration's rules.

Even more, health care's market bureaucracy amasses equally within the walls of private industry (McMaken 2015). The exchanges rely on private insurer participation, and their costs of operating, including high profits and salaries, is part of the cost of the market-based bureaucracy. It is unsurprising that the administrative costs of the US health care system well outpace those of its peers (Frakt 2018).

Furthermore, the exchanges have commanded oversized technocratic analysis of their successes and shortcomings, consuming the time and energy of talented researchers and think tanks. Scholars, news outlets, and policy makers obsess over every twist and turn, from an insurer joining or dropping out to the ups and downs of premium prices. The *New York Times* alone published over 300 articles on the ACA exchanges from 2010 to 2016 (Hoffman 2019b).

The result is a market-lubricating regulatory scaffold—a bureaucracy perhaps larger than what a direct regulatory approach would produce, and equally vulnerable to capture, or perhaps even more so because, by definition, private industry holds the reins to success. Yet, this expensive tinkering provides insurance for a mere 3% of the population and sets them up to make poor plan choices.

The ACA perpetuates health care's market bureaucracy, yet it is only a small part of it. Managed competition has equally informed the design of the Medicare supplemental market, including Medicare Advantage, Medigap, and the Medicare Part D market. Beyond insurance, an equally futile market bureaucracy grew from consumer-driven approaches to medical care choices. There regulatory scaffolding supports policies attempting with little success to incentivize patients to make good choices to reduce their use of low-value care or to find lower-priced providers (Hoffman 2019b). Likewise, modern antitrust regulation attempts, also with little success, to generate market dynamics that will drive higher-value health care. As antitrust expert Thomas Greaney (2009: 225) described, "Properly applied, antitrust law should promote decentralized decision-making by market participants while encouraging efficient combinations that serve consumer welfare." These policies all privilege market choice

---

3. CMS n.d. counts listings under "Health Insurance Marketplaces" through calendar year 2016.

and dynamics to achieve larger health policy goals. In turn, regulatory structures focus on scaffolding, lubricating, and repairing markets that in theory will enable people to choose what they value most, even though this theory repeatedly falls short in application.

The ACA has continued to build the market bureaucracy. Although 20 million more Americans now have health insurance, about half through the exchanges, the ACA arguably paved a painful and expensive path to this end.

The Sociological Problem with Choice of Health Plan

The market bureaucracy, in turn, feeds a modern American obsession with choice. Pouring effort into regulatory structures aimed at bolstering choice perpetuates the idea that choice should be the ultimate goal.

This veneration of choice as *the* American value has been building since at least the 1960s. Early kernels in health care might be traced to reproductive and civil rights activists, and legal cases like *Griswold v. Connecticut* in 1965 (381 U.S. 479, 483) and *Roe v. Wade* in 1973 (410 U.S. 113, 170), which favored individual control through a language prohibiting government intrusion over individual reproductive choices. Choice defined the early disability rights movement and demands for independent living and self-direction instead of institutionalization (Administration for Community Living, n.d.). It echoes in works like *Our Bodies Ourselves*, published in 1970 by the Boston Women's Health Collaborative, seeking to help women find self-empowerment over their bodies (Our Bodies, Our Selves, n.d.).

In health care, the sanctification of choice is in part a reaction to a system in which what patients wanted long came second. For most of the twentieth century, doctors controlled medical care decisions. Then, central planning and managed care emerged to address high spending in the 1970s and 1980s, and regulators and insurers gained decisional control. When those efforts fell short, consumer choice grew as something of a "sacred value" (Tetlock 2003). Informed consent evolved and aimed to put medical decisions back in the hands of patients. Market-based policies grew up in parallel, which elevated individual choice, defined by buying power.

Yet, this veneration of choice has arguably gone too far. A world of increasing market choices is actively making people worse off (Schwartz 2004). Not only do people often make poor choices, but people also dread making choices. Thirty percent of respondents to one survey reported they would rather prepare their taxes than navigate health insurance (eHealthinsurance 2008). The very existence of a market-based system can be contrary to what makes people, at least some people, feel better off. One study revealed that, although the idea of choice was associated with positive attributes for middle-class respondents, working-class respondents associated it with negative attributes and difficulty (Stephens, Fryberg, and Markus 2011).

Choice can also obfuscate what people collectively value and impede productive policies. Studies show that activating the idea of choice can decrease support for policies promoting equality and societal benefits (Savani, Stephens, and Markus 2011). The ACA offers an illustration of this idea. Although it might have been otherwise (Hoffman 2011), the downfall of the ACA's individual mandate came in part because it sought to achieve a collective goal through individual action. It prompted Americans to focus on their own bottom line—exactly how much an insurance policy cost and what it provided in return—instead of on the goal of universal access to health care. Choice centered the policy discussion in the wrong ideological place. The ACA's health insurance reforms make this same mistake more broadly. They elevate the idea that choice of health plan is in and of itself an important goal. In turn, regulatory efforts futilely attempt to achieve this goal, without question.

Yet, at the end of the day, most Americans do not care if their insurance comes from Aetna or Blue Cross. Many people do not know their own plan deductible—if they know what a deductible is—and many would struggle to weigh a choice between a plan with a $10 copay or 10% coinsurance. Most people do, however, care about access to good doctors and hospitals. And Americans do care that they and others can get access to necessary health care without going broke. The most important collective goals may have very little to do with choice, and it will be necessary to move choice aside to understand this reality.

The Post-ACA Horizon for Choice

As the ACA turns 10, we can celebrate that it brought deep national attention to the goal of universal coverage, even if it has not yet achieved it. It also provides a moment to reflect on whether choice should remain the guiding light going forward.

As candidates gear up for the 2020 election, they risk perpetuating the reverence of choice. Candidates who want to build on the ACA's infrastructure sell choice, advocating for a public option for more choice. Perhaps most evident, Pete Buttigieg called for "Medicare for all who want it." He asserted that if Medicare is the best option, people will choose it, and it will slowly displace inferior private plans. Vice President Joe Biden calls for "giving Americans a new choice, a public health insurance option like Medicare." (Biden for President 2019).

Part of why these candidates sell choice is to differentiate themselves from advocates for a single-payer plan. Choice serves as a euphemistic promise to enfranchised Americans with gold-plated health insurance to let them keep their plans, as well as a balm to others who are loyal to their plans, whether their plans deserve such loyalty or not, or who are fearful of change. Candidates know and bank on the resonance of choice among voters—a resonance crafted through years of careful public-relations campaigns by opponents to single-payer health care (Potter 2020)—even among candidates who understand that choice is a largely empty promise. Proponents of Medicare for All also reinforce the centrality of choice, either by selling this idea based on choice of doctor, which Medicare for All would enhance for many people, or by crafting transition plans that look like opting into Medicare for All.

Choice keeps its stronghold in part based on the narrative that what Americans want is too heterogeneous to be captured by any one solution. Yet, even at this moment when democracy limps along, democratic deliberation over health care priorities is vibrant, and sometimes reveals shared ground. Without overemphasizing the extent of such shared ground since Americans are clearly divided on many critical aspects of health policy, the places of shared commitments could suggest a basis for policy-making priorities. For example, widespread outrage over exorbitant drug pricing and the bind in which it has put many American families is clear. Americans identified lowering drug prices as a top 2017 congressional priority (Council of Economic Advisers 2018). Likewise, in the summer of 2017, public outcry arose against the newly elected Republican Congress's effort to repeal the ACA (Sessions, Cassidy, and Goodman 2017), suggesting at least high-level support for greater access.

The fight over Medicaid expansion reinforces this theme. The ACA intended to require states to expand Medicaid access to anyone earning up to 138% of the federal poverty level, but the ACA's first major legal challenge, *NFIB v. Sebelius*, effectively made this expansion optional. As of September 2018, 34 states and the District of Columbia had expanded (Kaiser Family Foundation 2018).

In the more conservative opt-out states, voters have begun to directly override their representatives' decision not to expand Medicaid in these states through ballot initiatives (Antoinisse and Rudowitz 2019). Maine passed a ballot initiative to expand Medicaid in November 2017 and voters in Idaho, Nebraska, and Utah followed in November 2018. These ballot initiatives suggest that voters value access to medical care in their communities, especially for lower-income community members. For these initiatives to pass required people who would not directly benefit personally to vote in favor. When the populace expresses shared commitments, whether in abstract terms like valuing access or concrete terms like lower drug prices, it is the job of elected representatives to overcome political barriers to respond. Yet, to the contrary and reflective of deep political dysfunction, legislatures and governors in Medicaid ballot-initiative states dig in their heels deeper to resist expansion, and Congress stalls out again and again on drug pricing reforms. We then turn futilely back to markets with the hope that they will fix the things that our politicians are increasingly unable and unwilling to fix.

Bureaucracy is inevitable, but it should bolster a health care system that can fulfill, rather than frustrate, what people and communities genuinely care about. Looking slightly under the surface suggests that what people really care most about is not always choice and that it is time to refocus health regulation on realizing other shared values.

▪ ▪ ▪

Allison K. Hoffman is professor of law at University of Pennsylvania Carey Law School and senior fellow at Penn's Leonard Davis Institute of Health Economics. Her work questions the role of regulation and the welfare state in promoting health and wellbeing as well as how regulation affects conceptions of risk and responsibility. ahoffman@law.upenn.edu

References

Abaluck, Jason, and Jonathan Gruber. 2011. "Heterogeneity in Choice Inconsistencies among the Elderly: Evidence from Prescription Drug Plan Choice." *American Economic Review* 101, no. 3: 377–381.

Administration for Community Living. 2019. "About Community Living." April 23. acl.gov/about-community-living.

Afendulis, Christopher C., Anna D. Sinaiko, and Richard G. Frank. 2015. "Dominated Choices and Medicare Advantage Enrollment." *Journal of Economic Behavior and Organization* 119: 72–83.

Antoinisse, Larisa, and Robin Rudowitz. 2019. "An Overview of State Approaches to Adopting the Medicaid Expansion." Kaiser Family Foundation, February 27. www.kff.org/report-section/an-overview-of-state-approaches-to-adopting-the-medicaid-expansion-issue-brief/.

Avalere Health. 2015. "More Than 2 Million Exchange Enrollees Forgo Cost-Sharing Assistance." August 19. avalere.com/expertise/managed-care/insights/more-than-2-million-exchange-enrollees-forgo-cost-sharing-assistance.

Barnes, Andrew J., Yaniv Hanoch, and Thomas Rice. 2014. "Determinants of Coverage Decisions in Health Insurance Marketplaces: Consumers' Decision-Making Abilities and the Amount of Information in their Choice Environment." *Health Services Research* 50, no. 1: 58–80.

Bhargava, Saurabh, and George Loewenstein. 2015. "Choosing a Health Insurance Plan: Complexity and Consequences." *JAMA* 314, no. 23: 2505–6.

Bhargava, Saurabh, George Loewenstein, and Shlomo Benartzi. 2017. "The Costs of Poor Health (Plan Choices) and Prescriptions for Reform." *Behavioral Science and Policy* 3, no. 1: 1–14.

Bhargava, Saurabh, George Loewenstein, and Justin Sydnor. 2017. "Choose to Lose: Health Plan Choices from a Menu with Dominated Options." *Quarterly Journal of Economics* 132, no. 3: 1319–72.

Biden for President. 2019. "Health Care." joebiden.com/healthcare/ (accessed February 10, 2020).

CBO (Congressional Budget Office). 2010. "CBO's August 2010 Baseline: Health Insurance Exchanges." August 25. www.cbo.gov/sites/default/files/111th-congress-2009-2010/dataandtechnicalinformation/ExchangesAugust2010FactSheet.pdf.

CMS (Centers for Medicare and Medicaid). n.d. "The Center for Consumer Information and Insurance Oversight: Regulations and Guidance." www.cms.gov/CCIIO/Resources/Regulations-and-Guidance/index.html#HealthInsurance Marketplaces (accessed February 6, 2020).

Council of Economic Advisers. 2018. "CEA Report: Reforming Biopharmaceutical Pricing at Home and Abroad." White House, February 9. www.whitehouse.gov/briefings-statements/cea-report-reforming-biopharmaceutical-pricing-home-abroad/.

Covered California. 2018. "Proposed Fiscal Year 2018–2019 Budget." May 17. board.coveredca.com/meetings/2018/05-17/CoveredCA_2018-19_Proposed_Budget-5-17-18.pdf.

Dafny, Leemore S. 2014. "Hospital Industry Consolidation—Still More to Come?" *New England Journal of Medicine* 370, no. 3: 198–99.

eHealth. 2008. "New Survey Shows Americans Lack Understanding of Their Health Coverage and Basic Health Insurance Terminology." January 3. news.ehealthinsurance.com/news/rel344367.

Enthoven, Alain C. 1978a. "Consumer-Choice Health Plan (First of Two Parts). Inflation and Inequity in Health Care Today: Alternatives for Cost Control and an Analysis of Proposals for National Health Insurance." *New England Journal of Medicine* 298, no. 12: 650–58.

Enthoven, Alain C. 1978b. "Consumer Choice Health Plan (Second of Two Parts). A National-Health Insurance Proposal Based on Regulated Competition in the Private Sector." *New England Journal of Medicine* 298, no. 13: 709–20.

Enthoven, Alain C. 1993. "The History and Principles of Managed Competition." *Health Affairs* 25, no. 1: 24–48.

Frakt, Austin. 2018. "The Astonishingly High Administrative Costs of U.S. Health Care." *New York Times*, July 16. www.nytimes.com/2018/07/16/upshot/costs-health -care-us.html.

Fung, Vicki et al. 2017. "Nearly One-Third of Enrollees in California's Individual Market Missed Opportunities to Receive Financial Assistance." *Health Affairs* 36, no. 1: 21–31.

Garnick, Deborah W., Ann Hendricks, Ken Thorpe, Joe Newhouse, Karen Donelan, and Bob Blendon. 1993. "How Well Do Americans Understand Their Health Coverage?" *Health Affairs* 12, no. 3: 204–12.

Gaynor, Martin, and Robert Town. 2012. "The Impact of Hospital Consolidation— Update." Robert Wood Johnson Foundation, June. www.rwjf.org/en/library /research/2012/06/the-impact-of-hospital-consolidation.html.

Glied, Sherry A. M. 2007. "Comments on Enthoven's 'The US Experience with Managed Care and Managed Competition.'" In *Wanting It All: The Challenge of Reforming the US Health Care System*, edited by J. Sneddon Little, 127–34. Boston: Federal Reserve Bank of Boston.

Greaney, Thomas. 2009. "Competition Policy and Organizational Fragmentation in Health Care." *University of Pittsburgh Law Review* 71, no. 2: 217–39.

Heiss, Florian, Adam Leive, Daniel McFadden, and Joachim Winter. 2012. "Plan Selection in Medicare Part D: Evidence from Administrative Data." NBER Working Paper 18166, National Bureau of Economic Research, June. www.nber .org/papers/w18166.

Hoffman, Allison K. 2011. "Oil and Water: Mixing Individual Mandates, Fragmented Markets, and Health Reform." *American Journal of Law and Medicine* 36, no. 1: 7–77.

Hoffman, Allison K. 2019a. "Cost-Sharing Reductions, Technocratic Tinkering, and Market-Based Health Policy." *Journal of Law, Medicine, and Ethics* 46: 873–76.

Hoffman, Allison K. 2019b. Forthcoming. "Health Care's Market Bureaucracy." *UCLA Law Review* 66.

Johnson, Eric J., Ran Hassin, Tom Baker, Allison T. Bajger, and Galen Treuer. 2013. "Can Consumers Make Affordable Care Affordable? The Value of Choice Architecture." *PLOS ONE* 8, no. e81521: 1–6.

Kahneman, Daniel, and Amos Tversky. 1979. "Prospect Theory: An Analysis of Decision under Risk." *Econometrica* 47, no. 2: 263–92.

Kaiser Family Foundation. 2018. "Status of State Action on the Medicaid Expansion Decision." State Health Facts, September 18. www.kff.org/health-reform/state -indicator/state-activity-around-expanding-medicaid-under-the-affordable-care-act /?currentTimeframe=0&sortModel=%7B%22colId%22:%22Location%22,%22 sort%22:%22asc%22%7D.

Kaiser Family Foundation. 2019. "Marketplace Enrollment 2014–2019." State Health Facts. www.kff.org/health-reform/state-indicator/marketplace-enrollment/?current Timeframe=0&sortModel=%7B%22colId%22:%22Location%22,%22sort%22:% 22asc%22%7D (accessed February 10, 2020).

Koma, Wyatt, Juliette Cubanski, Gretchen Jacobson, Anthony Damico, and Tricia Neuman. 2019. "No Itch to Switch: Few Medicare Beneficiaries Switch Plans during the Open Enrollment Period." Kaiser Family Foundation, December 2. www.kff.org/medicare/issue-brief/no-itch-to-switch-few-medicare-beneficiaries -switch-plans-during-the-open-enrollment-period/.

Loewenstein, George, Joelle Y. Friedman, Barbara McGill, Sarah Ahmad, Suzanne Linck, Stacey Sidula, John Beshears, et al. 2013. "Consumers' Misunderstanding of Health Insurance." *Journal of Health Economics* 32, no. 5: 850–62.

Mach, Annie L., and C. Stephen Redhead. 2014. "Federal Funding for Health Insurance Exchanges." Congressional Research Services, October 19. www.fas.org/sgp /crs/misc/R43066.pdf; perma.cc/GPD6–RNDX.

Marone, James A. 1994. "Neglected Institutions: Politics, Administration, and Health Reform." *Political Science and Politics* 27, no. 2: 220–23.

McMaken, Ryan. 2015. "'Social Expenditures' in the US Are Higher than All Other Countries, Except France." *Mises Wire*, October 30. mises.org/wire/social-expen ditures-us-are-higher-all-other-oecd-countries-except-france.

Nelson, Wendy, Valerie F. Reyna, Angela Fagerlin, Isaac Lipkus, and Ellen Peters. 2008. "Clinical Implications of Numeracy: Theory and Practice." *Annals of Behavioral Medicine* 35, no. 3: 261–74.

Our Bodies, Our Selves. n.d. "Our Story." www.ourbodiesourselves.org/our-story (accessed February 8, 2020).

Peters, Ellen, and Irwin P. Levin. 2008. "Dissecting the Risky-Choice Framing Effect: Numeracy as an Individual-Difference Factor in Weighing Risky and Riskless Options." *Judgment and Decision Making* 3, no. 6: 435–48.

Potter, Wendell. 2020. "How the Health Insurance Industry (and I) Invented the 'Choice' Talking Point." *New York Times*, January 14. www.nytimes.com/2020/01 /14/opinion/healthcare-choice-democratic-debate.html.

Reyna, Valerie F., Wendy L. Nelson, Paul K. Han, and Nathan F. Dieckman. 2009. "How Numeracy Influences Risk Comprehension and Medical Decision Making." *Psychological Bulletin* 135, no. 6: 943–73.

Savani, Krishna, Nicole M. Stephens, and Hazel Rose Markus. 2011. "The Unanticipated Interpersonal and Society Consequences of Choice: Victim Blaming and Reduced Support for the Public Good." *Psychological Science* 22, no. 6: 795–802.

Schwartz, Barry. 2004. *The Paradox of Choice*. New York: Harper Perennial.

Sessions, Pete, Bill Cassidy, and John C. Goodman. 2017. "How We Can Repeal the ACA and Still Insure the Uninsured." *Health Affairs*, January 18. www.health affairs.org/do/10.1377/hblog20170118.058364/full/#one.

Sinaiko, Anna D., and Richard A. Hirth. 2011. "Consumers, Health Insurance, and Dominated Choices." *Journal of Health Economics* 30, no. 2: 450–57.

Stephens, Nicole M., Stephanie A. Fryberg, and Hazel Rose Markus. 2011. "When Choice Does Not Equal Freedom: A Sociocultural Analysis of Agency in Working-Class American Contexts." *Social, Psychological, and Personality Science* 2, no. 1: 33–41.

Tetlock, Philip E. 2003. "Thinking the Unthinkable: Sacred Values and Taboo Cognitions." *Trends in Cognitive Sciences* 7, no. 7: 320–24.

Vogel, Steven K. 2018. *Marketcraft: How Governments Make Markets Work*. Oxford: Oxford University Press.

Vogt, William B., and Robert Town. 2006. *How Has Hospital Consolidation Affected the Price and Quality of Hospital Care?* Princeton, NJ: Robert Wood Johnson Foundation.

Weinstein, Neil D. 1980. "Unrealistic Optimism about Future Life Events." *Journal of Personality and Social Psychology* 39, no. 5: 806–20.

The Secretary Shall . . . : Implementing the Affordable Care Act's Private Insurance Expansions

Sherry Glied
New York University

Aryana Khalid
Marilyn B. Tavenner

Abstract The federal bureaucracy played a critical role in implementing most aspects of the Affordable Care Act's private insurance coverage expansion. Through brief case studies, the authors review three dimensions of this role: the development of the Center for Consumer Information and Insurance Oversight, rulemaking in the formulation of the essential health benefits package, and the implementation of the federal website. They relate these to themes in the public administration literature. Politics—both through state decisions and through continuing congressional action (and inaction)—pervaded the implementation process. The challenges of staffing and situating the new bureaucracy effectively changed vertical boundaries within the Department of Health and Human Services, with long-lasting consequences. Finally, the complex design of the policy itself made passage of the legislation easier but implementation much more difficult. Ultimately, however, implementation was remarkably successful, achieving improvements in coverage consistent with the Congressional Budget Office's projections.

Keywords Affordable Care Act, implementation, public management

The Affordable Care Act (ACA) passed on March 23, 2010. By 2015, the number of Americans with health insurance had increased by over 20 million (Zammitti, Cohen, and Martinez 2016). Tens of millions more had seen improvements in the scope and quality of their coverage. Through the ACA, Congress appropriated the funds, authorized the taxes, and described the rules that led to these changes. But the ACA also required substantial executive action, in the form of new regulations governing the behavior of others and in operationalizing new programs, to have actual effect. The

Journal of Health Politics, Policy and Law, Vol. 45, No. 4, August 2020
DOI 10.1215/03616878-8255457   © 2020 by Duke University Press

ACA reads "The Secretary shall" 1,563 times (Conover and Ellig 2012). Each of those "shalls" required someone in the executive branch of government to do something. The ACA appropriated $1 billion to cover internal government costs for all this "doing."

Many important elements of the ACA were modifications of existing programs. The ACA made important changes to Medicare payment methodologies and benefits. Much of the coverage expansion in the law occurred through Medicaid. These Medicare and Medicaid changes required enormous effort and often substantial creativity on the part of the federal bureaucracy, but they fit into established structures. Medicare had changed payment methods and expanded benefits before. Medicaid eligibility had been expanded over time, and the rules governing eligibility had changed. While these reforms and expansions touched thousands of providers and millions of people, it is testimony to the strengths of the federal administrative system that modifications of this scope and scale can be considered part of the "normal science" of federal programs.

Many of the elements of the ACA, however, involved incursions of the federal government into areas where there had been little prior federal presence. Most significant of these were changes made to the rules governing private insurance, the design of nongroup insurance benefits, and the establishment of health insurance exchanges. As Brown (1983) described in the case of the implementation of the 1973 HMO Act, this early implementation process can be decomposed into discrete organizational tasks: the development of a new bureaucracy, rulemaking, and implementation. In the next section of this article, we briefly describe these three sets of activities. In the final section, we consider broader questions they raise about policy implementation.

Organization: The Evolution of the Center for Consumer Information and Insurance Oversight

The ACA's regulation of private health insurance had two sets of components. One group of components was intended to be permanent and to lay the groundwork for the transformed health insurance market that would become fully operational with the opening of the Exchanges (later Marketplaces) in 2014. These included regulations governing medical loss ratios, coverage of dependents, elimination of annual and lifetime limits on covered expenses, and risk adjustment rules. The second group of components were intended as stop-gap measures that would remain in place only until the exchanges opened. These components—now virtually forgotten—included the Pre-existing Condition Insurance Plan, a set of high-risk pools operating in each state; elimination of preexisting condition exclusions for children; an early retiree reinsurance program; and an informational website that displayed current insurance prices in the non-group market.

Most of these activities were federal extensions of activities that had long been undertaken by state insurance regulators. The ACA's rules in this sphere were largely intended to be implemented through state insurance commissioners, with the goal of increasing the consistency of insurance regulation across the country.

The Secretary of the Department of Health and Human Services (HHS), Kathleen Sebelius, had extensive experience in private insurance (having served as insurance commissioner prior to becoming governor of Kansas). Outside the secretary's office, however, HHS's familiarity with private insurance was limited to the Medicare Advantage and Part D drug programs, which posed their own challenges but were relatively circumscribed and addressed a known population. Because of the secretary's expertise, and the expectation that HHS's role would be largely limited to working with states to implement a set of consistent regulations, HHS initially assigned responsibility for private insurance regulation to a new office reporting to the secretary, the Office of Consumer Information and Insurance Oversight (OCIIO), and hired another former insurance commissioner to lead this office (GAO 2013).

OCIIO, unlike a typical state insurance regulator, would, in many cases, be adopting regulations that governed both state insurance markets (plans not exempt from the Employee Retirement Income Security Act of 1974 [ERISA]) and parts of the health insurance market that fell outside those bounds. Operationally, this meant that, in addition to HHS, the Department of Labor, which regulates self-insured/ERISA plans, and the Department of the Treasury, which regulates tax-favored health programs (such as health savings accounts), would need to work together to develop all regulations. Given the political salience of the ACA and the need to coordinate efforts across departments, the White House held meetings twice a week in the Eisenhower Executive Office Building with the principals from each of the agencies responsible for implementing the ACA, to ensure this coordination. The $1 billion in implementation funding would need to be divided fairly across all these agencies.

This might have been a recipe for serious interdepartmental strain. In practice, while there were certainly vigorous debates in the Eisenhower Building, there was remarkable consensus about the need to move forward, partly in response to mounting partisan opposition. Notably, over the entire period between passage of the law and the opening of the marketplaces, there were no significant media leaks about the content of upcoming regulations or about internal disagreements. Nonetheless, the need to work collaboratively across three departments absorbed considerable time and energy.

The second set of challenges emerged in the regulation of new markets, where the evidence base was limited. For example, available surveys of annual limits in health insurance plans asked only whether such limits were below $250,000 (National Archives 2010). The promulgation of regulations governing these annual limits revealed the existence of millions of "bare-bones" insurance policies, with annual limits in the single- or double-digit thousands of dollars. OCIIO had to develop and implement a contentious emergency waiver process to hold together these shabby policies until 2014.

The first year of regulatory activities made it clear to HHS that the human and fiscal resources needed to implement the ACA would be far greater than anticipated. The programmatic challenges were magnified by partisan opposition to the ACA at the federal, state, and public level, which hardened over time. Congress had appropriated substantial funding for states to implement insurance regulations and to build their own state-based exchanges. While initially most states cooperated with OCIIO in standardizing regulations, such as rate review, and all but one had accepted funding to begin building exchanges, over time cooperation waned, with many states choosing not to build their own exchanges and returning grant funding (Fulton et al. 2015; Gluck and Huberfeld 2018; Jones 2017; Jones, Bradley, and Oberlander 2014).

The election of a Republican House majority in 2010 meant that further funding for implementation of the ACA was unlikely, though estimated implementation costs were 5–10 times higher than the $1 billion appropriated (Levinson 2016). In the face of these challenges, in early 2011 the secretary made the decision to move OCIIO into the Centers for Medicare and Medicaid Services (CMS), where it was renamed the Center for Consumer Information and Insurance Oversight (CCIIO). By moving OCIIO into CMS, the secretary could achieve economies of scale using CMS's expertise in the regulatory process, contracting, management, resources, and technical support (Gogan, Davidson, and Proudfoot 2016).

Writing the Rules: Essential Health Benefits

Section 1302(b) of the ACA calls on the secretary of HHS to define the scope of essential health benefits (EHBs) that shall be made available to those obtaining insurance coverage in the new marketplaces. The law specifies 10 broad categories of benefits that must be included in the EHBs; it limits the scope of these benefits, requiring that they equal those in the "typical employer plan"; and it adds a grab-bag list of considerations for the secretary in developing the EHBs. In addition, section 1311(d)(3) of the ACA allows states to mandate the inclusion of benefits in addition to those in the federal EHBs but requires that states defray the cost of any such benefits. Beyond its vaguely worded limitations and requirements, the ACA offers little in the way of specificity around these benefits.

The EHBs would form the basis of insurer's bids in the new market-places. The ACA's provision calling on states to pay for the costs of mandates that exceeded the scope of the EHB contemplated further state legislative action to repeal such mandates. The regulatory process for developing and releasing a final regulation would take at least 6 months. To give states and insurers time to act in time for the January 1, 2014, start date for the marketplaces, HHS would need to have a well-defined idea of the scope of the EHB before late 2011 (Bagley and Levy 2014).

The administration proceeded along three parallel paths to meet this timetable and objective. First, in the fall of 2010 the Office of the Secretary contracted with the Institute of Medicine (IOM) to convene an expert panel and deliver a consensus report recommending a process for defining the initial benefit package and for updating the benefit package over time. Second, the Department of Labor began its analysis of data from the National Compensation Survey on the scope of benefits in "typical" plans. Finally, the HHS heard from various interest groups with views on the regulations.

The IOM released its initial report in early October 2011 (see Ulmer et al. 2012). It recommended that the secretary begin with a small employer plan, add benefits to round out the 10 categories required by the law, and then trim benefits to hold the overall cost of the package to the cost of a typical plan. It suggested that HHS engage in a structured, deliberative process of soliciting public input, through a series of small-group meetings, to further prioritize services within the plan. Finally, the IOM proposed that a national board update the benefits over time, adding and subtracting benefits to hold costs to a premium target.

This proposal raised serious political and logistical hurdles. The administration was struggling with vehement political opposition to the ACA's Independent Payment Advisory Board, and the idea of proposing another board that could be tarred as a "death panel" to determine benefits before the critical 2012 elections was unrealistic (Spatz 2011). In addition, the proposal's target premium idea, designed to encourage states to drop costly mandates, would put tremendous pressure on states at a time when the administration was trying to encourage them to expand Medicaid and establish marketplaces. Finally, the small-group deliberative process was incompatible with the timetable for releasing benefits.

The Department of Labor's analysis of its existing survey data provided even less granularity than expected about the scope of benefits. Examination of plan documents specifying benefits was similarly unilluminating. There turned out to be relatively little variation across markets in the principle elements of plans. Differences among plans emerged in access to a limited number of specific services: bariatric surgery, infertility treatment, chiropractic, hearing aids, and autism treatment (Skopec et al. 2011; Uberoi 2015).

The three paths yielded very little insight about how to proceed. Fortunately, after the ACA passed, one of the lead finance committee staffers who had subsequently joined the administration suggested a way out: build on the model used for the State Children's Health Insurance Program. Under this program, states could choose a benefit package from a menu of existing choices offered to state and federal employees. This approach avoided the messy work of weighing one benefit against another. Given the law's requirement that benefits reflect a typical plan, and the IOM's recommendation that benefits reflect a small, rather than large, employer plan, HHS added the three largest small employer plans in the state to the menu of options. This extension had the added feature that most state mandates applied to small employer plans. That meant that if a state chose a small employer plan as the basis of its EHB, all existing state mandates would fall within the scope of the EHB, and the state would neither have to pay the cost of these mandates nor repeal them. Given the partisan rancor around the ACA, the administration anticipated that some states would not make an EHB selection and designated the largest small employer plan in the state (which would generally incorporate state mandates) as the default (CCIIO 2011).

The "menu" idea solved many problems, but it was completely outside the bounds of what anyone had expected, especially because there had been no press leaks signaling that the menu approach was a direction under consideration (Bagley and Levy 2014). The requirements of the federal rulemaking process meant that if HHS released the proposal as a Notice of Proposed Rulemaking (NPRM), there would need to be an extended comment period and a formal process of revision and response. The administration worried that there might be a fundamental flaw to the idea, in which case following the NPRM process would be fatal to the exchange launch timetable. After extensive consultation with the Office of the General Counsel, the HHS decided to take the unorthodox step of releasing a bulletin describing the idea in December 2011 (Bagley and Levy 2014).

Reactions to the bulletin were generally positive, praising the choice as "a deft political move" (Levey 2012) or grudgingly accepting, given the political constraints (Sage 2011). The HHS released an NPRM governing the collection of data to establish the menu in June 2012; an NPRM on the scope of EHBs in late November 2012, after the 2012 election; and a final rule on February 20, 2013, well after state and insurer decisions on exchanges had been made.

Building the Federal Marketplace

A component of the ACA legislation required the development of marketplaces—consumer-facing website(s) that would allow qualified individuals to "sign up" for insurance electronically. The federal website, HealthCare.gov, went live on October 1, 2013, to worldwide media attention, in the midst of a government shutdown. On that first day, only six people were able to enroll, as the website crashed. Only by early December, after a harrowing, costly, and massive intervention, did the website work properly (Levinson 2016). While the initial failure of the website had only modest impacts on the number of people who signed up for coverage in the first enrollment period, it took a considerable political toll (GAO 2015; Levinson 2016; Light 2014; Polsky, Weiner, and Becker 2014a).

The website comprised two quite distinct information technology (IT) platforms. First, on the front end, there would need to be a consumer-friendly website that allowed an individual to shop for Medicaid or private insurance. Second, on the back end, this consumer-facing website would need to access a great deal of highly confidential federal data (citizenship or immigration status, tax returns, identity through social security, and eligibility for other health care programs) to verify eligibility for private coverage, subsidies, and Medicaid. This back end became known as the "Hub."

The ACA had contemplated that each state would establish its own consumer-facing website, integrated with its Medicaid programs, and Congress had appropriated funds for this purpose. CCIIO would need to develop regulations governing the functioning of these state websites, including the application form for insurance, and protocols for the interaction between these state-level sites and the Hub.

There would be a single Hub for the federal and state-based market-places, operated by CCIIO in collaboration with the various agencies to be queried. Funding for the Hub was intended to come out of the $1 billion appropriation. The front-end, consumer-facing websites would need to collect the extensive information needed to verify eligibility through the Hub.

Most observers had presumed that states, which had regulatory authority over insurance, would want to manage their own exchanges (Levinson 2016). Initially, all but one sought and received an exchange grant for that purpose, with $3.6 billion in exchange planning grants dispersed (Gluck and Huberfeld 2018). As the ACA litigation progressed, several Republican-led states pulled back for political reasons, returning their planning grants (Gluck and Huberfeld 2018). The technical challenges of building a consumer-facing website deterred others (Vestal and Ollove 2013). Thus, by the time states were required to certify the operation of the website in early 2013 (a date that was delayed by HHS to encourage more states to participate), only 14 chose to proceed with their own designs, leaving HHS with responsibility for 37 consumer-facing websites, each linked to that individual state's Medicaid infrastructure (Dinan 2014; Gluck and Huberfeld 2018; Gogan, Davidson, and Proudfoot 2016; Noh 2016).

The development of the Hub seemed the more complex build, as it would require interfacing with varied IT systems across the federal government (GAO 2013), but the Hub has actually been a great unsung hero of federal technology development, as it has functioned nearly flawlessly since open enrollment in 2013. The front-end, consumer-facing websites ended up being the challenge, both for the federal government and for the states that chose to build their own sites. Ultimately, a total of 15 consumer-facing websites were built: one federal Marketplace and 14 state marketplaces (Vestal and Ollove 2013). Their varied experiences help shed light on the key problems. Ultimately, about one-third the state marketplaces ran smoothly from the outset; about one-third, including the federal Market-place, had a mixed performance in the first enrollment period; and about one-third had significant and enduring problems (Polsky, Weiner, and Becker 2014a, 2014b; Vestal and Ollove 2013). This variation in perfor-mance can be traced back to both design and contracting decisions (Fagnot, Ye, and Desouza 2018).

The first key design decision, which challenged the design of all the consumer-facing websites, was the application process. In its effort to exclude undocumented residents and to minimize crowd-out of existing insurance coverage, the law required a great deal of information about enrollees. Individuals seeking insurance could not be eligible for other forms of health care coverage (employer-sponsored insurance, unless the firm's offer of coverage was unaffordable; Medicare; Medicaid; or coverage through other federal programs) and had to be legal residents of the United States (GAO 2013). Income status and family size would further determine eligibility for subsidies or Medicaid.

Despite considerable efforts to simplify the collection of this information through the application process, it remained very complicated. The diversity of American families and their situations—new citizenship, adoptions, income fluctuations, employment shifts, and other variations—created a vast number of permutations to eligibility verification and subsidy calculation. These complexities could, in principle, be overcome, and the IT services company CGI Federal did conduct two successful demonstrations of the federal website in the weeks before launch (Levinson 2016). But such packaged demonstrations only showed that the system could handle complexity when inputs fell within expected parameters and the volume of queries was modest. At actual launch, multiple unanticipated permutations arose at high volume, applications were aborted, and, depending on system design, the strain on the website infrastructure became overwhelming.

The second key element was the contracting choice. In the case of the federal website, the set of potential vendors for the consumer-facing Marketplace contract was constrained by federal requirements; effectively choice was limited to contractors who had been prequalified years earlier. Ultimately, the contract was awarded to CGI Federal, which already had work under way within CMS (Gogan, Davidson, and Proudfoot 2016; Levinson 2016). In retrospect, CGI Federal's approach to the technical problem of building an exchange was likely flawed—the company was also the lead contractor for three of the least successful among the state exchanges: Hawaii, Massachusetts, and Vermont (Polsky et al. 2014a; Vestal and Ollove 2013). By contrast, the best-performing state exchanges (Connecticut, Kentucky, Rhode Island and Washington) were all contracted with Deloitte, which made a different set of web architecture and management decisions.

Finally, CMS (and some states), in the interest of getting the website finished in time, decided to delay the implementation of a "shopping" function beyond the open enrollment start. That decision meant that the hordes of people who were simply curious about the website but had no intention of buying coverage had to initiate a "fake" application to see the site. The flood of applications overwhelmed the site and led to the famous crash. Had shopping been available, visitors to the site would not have initiated an application process and there would have been less stress on the system.

The dramatic failure of the system led CMS, HHS, and the White House to mount a substantial rescue operation, which included shifting the technical work on the website from CGI Federal to QSSI, the contractor that had successfully built the Hub. CMS faced tremendous pressure to solve the problems. Contractors, IT experts, and staff worked 24/7 to solve the issues, even as a government shutdown limited the staff and resources available. The environment of 24/7 scrutiny by the media, Congress, advocates, and the White House unnerved everyone.

The key first step to righting the ship was introducing a shopping function, which took some burden off the application. Next, as the application support team gained experience, they were better able to help families with more complicated situations get through the process. Finally, CMS went through the painful process of identifying and solving IT bottlenecks and working a punch list. By January 2014 the number of people enrolled through the site had exceeded 1 million and the pressure eased.

Reflections

Several common themes flow across these three elements of ACA implementation, which had both short-term effects and long-term consequences.

Politics and Progress

The politics of the ACA clouded internal implementation efforts in several ways. Most obviously, state-level partisanship around Medicaid expansion and exchange establishment left the federal government with an unexpectedly large regulatory and implementation burden (Gluck and Huberfeld 2018; Oberlander 2016). But congressional politics also mattered. For example, exchange rules had to be in place in time for states to make decisions before January 2013. But the possibility that the Democrats might lose the Senate and presidency in 2012 pushed deadlines even further forward, out of fear that a new Congress would use the Congressional Review Act to nullify new regulations (Conover and Ellig 2012; Copeland and Beth 2008). In consequence, no substantial new HHS regulations were promulgated between late May 2012 and the elections that November, when the EHB NPRM was finally released.

The partisan shift in the House also interfered with the ability to manage the complex website contracts and regulatory processes, as congressional oversight intensified, with frequent requests for the secretary and CMS administrator to testify and enormous documentation requests, entangling the same staff tasked with regulatory development and coordination with insurers and states.

The ACA politics of 2010–14 continues to exert substantial influence on health care policy making. Most notably, a less partisan state environment might have led to the implementation of successful, state-managed, consumer-facing websites in more states, reinforcing the role of the states in future health reforms (Gluck and Huberfeld 2018).

Building a Bureaucracy

The short- and long-term success of a new public program depends on effectively drawing the vertical lines establishing and situating a new bureaucracy (Brown 1983; Kettl 2006). In sharp contrast to the evolution of a private-sector business, government bureaucracies do not arise spontaneously and grow incrementally. They must emerge from existing structures at scale, ready to serve tens of millions of customers on day one.

At the moment the ACA passed, HHS was already stretched thin managing ongoing programs and administering the rapid dispersal of over $17 billion in new American Recovery and Reinvestment Act Funds (Redhead et al. 2009). The day after the law passed, the Office of Personnel Management provided the HHS with direct hire authority, to facilitate hiring up to 1,480 people (Levinson 2016). However, relatively few people anywhere had the expertise needed to write the required new regulations; even fewer had experience working within the federal bureaucracy; still fewer had the ability to evaluate candidates for such positions. It had taken some 6–9 months to put staffing in place for the implementation of Medicare Part D back in 2003, and that was a much more bounded program within an existing infrastructure (Serafini 2010). The shortage of funding; endless oversight by the White House, Congress, and the media; and lucrative opportunities to work on state- and private-sector implementation of the law made it particularly challenging to recruit and retain effective senior-level managers within OCIIO. These funding and staffing challenges ultimately led to the move of OCIIO into the existing bureaucracy of CMS.

Integrating OCIIO into CCIIO stretched the role of the CMS administrator. Rather than acting as a quasi-apolitical manager administering well-established programs, the administrator's responsibilities now extended across the entire US health care system into the private sector. In this new structure, the recent clash between HHS Secretary Alex Azar and CMS Administrator Seema Verma over the future of the ACA may presage a series of battles to come (Pradhan, Cancryn, and Diamond 2019).

Policy Design and Execution

The design of the ACA itself posed significant challenges for implementation. The decision to generate immediate wins by starting transitional programs immediately (often with start dates of January 1, 2010, before the law had even passed) and then closing them out as new, permanent programs took their place proved to be very costly in terms of human resources (Conover and Ellig 2012). The transitory programs sprouted challenges of their own, requiring management and attracting congressional oversight.

The effort to constrain the costs of the program through the complex design of eligibility criteria meant that the website design became much more fraught. This wasn't building Travelocity—there was a sophisticated back-end eligibility system that had to accommodate permutations of the American family difficult to imagine. Ultimately, technical fixes saved the website. Computer designs today are quite capable of managing complex algorithms that include financial (means) testing and choices among dozens of insurance plan. But even the best computers don't eliminate the tensions inherent in the concurrent complexities of people's living situations and of choice-based program designs. The complexity of the ACA's design itself may be one source of the current interest in a conceptually simpler, non-means-tested, Medicare-for-all structure.

Implementation and Success

At the end of the day, the proof is in the pudding. Implementation of the ACA was far from perfect. Bugs big and small infected execution. The image of the HealthCare.gov website crashing is seared into the eyes of many health policy and management observers. But by the end of that first year, the US uninsurance rate had fallen by 7 percentage points, consistent with the Congressional Budget Office's projections at the time of enactment (Glied, Arora, and Solís-Román 2015; Zammitti, Cohen, and Martinez 2016). And as advocates had promised, Americans had better access to care and lower exposure to medical debt and bankruptcy. This tremendous historical success is owed, in large measure, to that much maligned institution, the federal bureaucracy.

■ ■ ■

Sherry Glied is dean of New York University's Robert F. Wagner Graduate School of Public Service. She was previously professor of health policy and management at Columbia University's Mailman School of Public Health. Between 2010 and 2012 she served as assistant secretary for planning and evaluation at the Department of Health and Human Services. She has been elected to the National Academy of Medicine and the National Academy of Social Insurance and served as a member of the Commission on Evidence-Based Policymaking. She holds a PhD in economics from Harvard University.
sherry.glied@nyu.edu

Aryana Khalid was chief of staff at the Centers for Medicare and Medicaid Services during most of the implementation of the Affordable Care Act. Before that she served as Senator Mark Warner's health and education legislative assistant. She also served as deputy secretary of health and human resources for the Commonwealth of Virginia for Governor Tim Kaine. She received her BS in systems engineering from the University of Virginia and her master of health administration from Virginia Commonwealth University. She currently lives in Malaysia and consults for US health care clients.

Marilyn B. Tavenner was appointed chief deputy of the Centers for Medicare and Medicaid Services (CMS) by the Obama administration in February 2010. She later served as CMS acting administrator and was confirmed as administrator by the Senate in 2013. In her 5 years at CMS she led the agency's implementation of the ACA. Before that she served as secretary of health in Virginia for Governor Tim Kaine. She received both her BS in nursing and her master in health administration from Virginia Commonwealth University.

Acknowledgments

We thank Aggie Tang for very useful research assistance. We thank the Commonwealth Fund for research support.

References

Bagley, Nicholas, and Helen Levy. 2014. "Essential Health Benefits and the Affordable Care Act: Law and Process." *Journal of Health Politics, Policy and Law* 39, no. 2: 441–65.

Brown, Lawrence D. 1983. *Politics and Health Care Organization.* Washington, DC: Brookings Institution.

CCIIO (Center for Consumer Information and Insurance Oversight). 2011. "Essential Health Benefits Bulletin." December 16. www.cms.gov/CCIIO/Resources/Files /Downloads/essential_health_benefits_bulletin.pdf.

Conover, Christopher J., and Jerry Ellig. 2012. "Beware the Rush to Presumption, Part C: A Public Choice Analysis of the Affordable Care Act's Interim Final Rules." Mercatus Center, January. www.mercatus.org/publications/regulation/beware-rush -presumption-part-c.

Copeland, Curtis W., and Richard S. Beth. 2008. "Congressional Review Act: Disapproval of Rules in a Subsequent Session of Congress." Congressional Research Service, September 3. fas.org/sgp/crs/misc/RL34633.pdf.

Dinan, John. 2014. "Implementing Health Reform: Intergovernmental Bargaining and the Affordable Care Act." *Publius* 44, no. 3: 399–425.

Fagnot, Isabelle, Chen Ye, and Kevin C. Desouza. 2018. "Unpacking Complexities of Mega-scale Public Sector Information Technology Projects: An Ecosystem Perspective." *Systèmes d'information et management* 23, no. 2: 9–41.

Fulton, Brent D., Ann Hollingshead, Pinar Karaca-Mandic, and Richard M. Scheffler. 2015. "Republican States Bolstered Their Health Insurance Rate Review Programs Using Incentives from the Affordable Care Act." *Inquiry* 52. doi.org/10.1177/ 0046958015604164.

GAO (Government Accountability Office). 2013. "Patient Protection and Affordable Care Act: Status of CMS Efforts to Establish Federally Facilitated Health Insurance Exchanges." June. www.gao.gov/assets/660/655291.pdf.

GAO (Government Accountability Office). 2015. "Healthcare.gov: CMS Has Taken Steps to Address Problems, but Needs to Further Implement Systems Development Best Practices." March. www.gao.gov/assets/670/668834.pdf.

Glied, Sherry A., Anupama Arora, and Claudia Solís-Román. 2015. "The CBO's Crystal Ball: How Well Did It Forecast the Effects of the Affordable Care Act?" Commonwealth Fund, December 15. www.commonwealthfund.org/publications /issue-briefs/2015/dec/cbos-crystal-ball-how-well-did-it-forecast-effects-affordable.

Gluck, Abbe R., and Nicole Huberfeld. 2018. "What Is Federalism in Healthcare For?" *Stanford Law Review* 70, no. 6: 1689.

Gogan, Janis L., Elizabeth J. Davidson, and Jeffrey Proudfoot. 2016. "The Health-Care.gov Project." *Journal of Information Technology Teaching Cases* 6, no. 2: 99–110.

Jones, David K. 2017. *Exchange Politics: Opposing Obamacare in Battleground States.* Oxford: Oxford University Press.

Jones, David K., Katherine W. V. Bradley, and Jonathan Oberlander. 2014. "Pascal's Wager: Health Insurance Exchanges, Obamacare, and the Republican Dilemma." *Journal of Health Politics, Policy and Law* 39, no. 1: 97–137.

Kettl, Donald F. 2006. "Managing Boundaries in American Administration: The Collaboration Imperative." *Public Administration Review* 66, no. s1: 10–19.

Levey, Noam N. 2012. "Passing the Buck—Or Empowering States? Who Will Define Essential Health Benefits." *Health Affairs* 31, no. 4: 663–66.

Levinson, Daniel R. 2016. "CMS Management of the Federal Marketplace: A Case Study." Department of Health and Human Services, Office of the Inspector General, February. oig.hhs.gov/oei/reports/oei-06-14-00350.pdf.

Light, Paul C. 2014. "A Cascade of Failures: Why Government Fails, and How to Stop It." Center for Effective Public Management, Brookings Institution, July. www .brookings.edu/research/a-cascade-of-failures-why-government-fails-and-how-to -stop-it/.

National Archives. 2010. "Patient Protection and Affordable Care Act: Preexisting Condition Exclusions, Lifetime and Annual Limits, Rescissions, and Patient Protections." *Federal Register*, June 28. www.federalregister.gov/documents/2010 /06/28/2010-15278/patient-protection-and-affordable-care-act-preexisting-condit ion-exclusions-lifetime-and-annual.

Noh, Shihyun. 2016. "Federal Strategies to Induce Resistant States to Participate in the ACA Health Exchanges." *State and Local Government Review* 48, no. 4: 227–35.

Oberlander, Jonathan. 2016. "Implementing the Affordable Care Act: The Promise and Limits of Health Care Reform." *Journal of Health Politics, Policy and Law* 41, no. 4: 803–26.

Polsky, Daniel E., Janet Weiner, Christopher Colameco, and Nora Becker. 2014a. "Deciphering the Data: Final Enrollment Rates Show Federally Run Marketplaces Make up Lost Ground at End of Enrollment." University of Pennsylvania Leonard Davis Institute of Health Economics and Robert Wood Johnson Foundation, May. ldi.upenn.edu/sites/default/files/pdf/final%20enrollment%20rates%20federal%20 marketplaces%20make%20up%20lost%20ground.pdf.

Polsky, Daniel, Janet Weiner, Christopher Colameco, and Nora Verlaine Becker. 2014b. "Health Insurance Marketplace Enrollment Rates by Type of Exchange." Data Brief, University of Pennsylvania Leonard Davis Institute of Health Economics, March 28. repository.upenn.edu/cgi/viewcontent.cgi?article=1010&context=ldi_databriefs.

Pradhan, Rachana, Adam Cancryn, and Dan Diamond. 2019. "Clashes among Top HHS Officials Undermine Trump Agenda." Politico, November 27. https://www .politico.com/news/2019/11/26/hhs-trump-azar-verma-074149.

Redhead, C. Stephen, Kirsten J. Colello, Sarah A. Lister, Bernice Reyes-Akinbileje, Pamela W. Smith, and Andrew R. Sommers. 2009. "Selected Health Funding in the American Recovery and Reinvestment Act." Congressional Research Service, February 20. crsreports.congress.gov/product/pdf/R/R40181.

Sage, William M. 2011. "CMS's Essential Benefits Guidance: Brush-Clearing or Can-Kicking?" *Health Affairs Blog*, December 28. www.healthaffairs.org/do/10.1377 /hblog20111228.015984/full/.

Serafini, Marilyn Werber. 2010. "Writing the Rules for the Health Law." *National Journal*, May 1: 6.

Skopec, Laura, Ashley Henderson, Susan Todd, and Pierre L. Yong. 2011. "Essential Health Benefits: Comparing Benefits in Small Group Products and State and Federal Employee Plans." Office of the Assistant Secretary for Planning and Evaluation, Office of Health Policy, Department of Health and Human Services, December. aspe.hhs.gov/system/files/pdf/180086/rb.pdf.

Spatz, Ian. 2011. "Defining Essential Benefits: Congress' Once and Future Role." *Health Affairs Blog*, February 17. www.healthaffairs.org/do/10.1377/hblog2011 0217.009354/full/.

Uberoi, Namrata K. 2015. "The Patient Protection and Affordable Care Act's Essential Health Benefits (EHB)." Congressional Research Service, August 27. fas.org/sgp /crs/misc/R44163.pdf.

Ulmer, Cheryl, John Ball, Elizabeth McGlynn, and Shadia Bel Hamdounia. 2012. *Essential Health Benefits: Balancing Coverage and Cost.* Washington, DC: National Academies Press.

Vestal, Christine, and Michael Ollove. 2013. "Why Some State-Run Health Exchanges Didn't Work." *Government Technology,* December 11. www.govtech.com/health /Why-Some-State-Run-Health-Exchanges-Didnt-Work.html.

Zammitti, Emily P., Robin A. Cohen, and Michael E. Martinez. 2016. "Health Insurance Coverage: Early Release of Estimates from the National Health Interview Survey, January–June 2016." National Health Interview Survey Early Release Program, National Center for Health Statistics, November. www.cdc.gov/nchs/data /nhis/earlyrelease/insur201611.pdf.

Promise, Performance, and Litigation

Lost in the ACA:
Bit Parts in a Landmark Law

John E. McDonough
Harvard University

Abstract The Affordable Care Act (ACA) is a mosaic across a spectrum of health policy domains. The law contains hundreds of smaller and mostly unnoticed reforms aimed at nearly every segment of American health policy. Ten years later, these provisions include successes, failures, and mixed bags, which should be considered in any full assessment of the ACA. This article examines 11 from each of these 3 categories, drawn from 9 of the ACA's 10 titles. These mininarratives deepen recognition that the ACA is our best example of comprehensive health reform and defies simplistic judgments.

Keywords Affordable Care Act

Though the Affordable Care Act (ACA) is only one law, the statute itself is a mosaic across a spectrum of health policy domains. Beside marquee provisions involving Medicare, Medicaid, private health insurance, delivery system transformation, and financing, the ACA contains hundreds of smaller and mostly unnoticed reforms aimed at nearly every segment of American health policy. Ten years later, these provisions include successes, failures, and mixed bags, which should be considered in any full assessment of the ACA. I examine 11, from each of these 3 categories, drawn from 9 of the ACA's 10 titles. These mininarratives deepen recognition that the ACA is our best example of comprehensive health reform and defies simplistic judgments.

The successes I examine comprise state-run health insurance exchanges, Medicaid's Modified Adjusted Gross Income (MAGI) standard, the Physician

Journal of Health Politics, Policy and Law, Vol. 45, No. 4, August 2020
DOI 10.1215/03616878-8255469   © 2020 by Duke University Press

Payments Sunshine Act, and new Medicare payroll taxes. Under proposed failures I examine health insurance cooperatives, the Independent Payment Advisory Board (IPAB), the Health Workforce Commission, and the Community Living Assistance Services and Supports (CLASS) program. Mixed results comprise Calorie Menu Labeling, the Elder Justice Act, and biosimilar biopharmaceutical innovation. For each, I describe what the enacted ACA component was intended to accomplish plus a summary of key developments since then. I conclude with brief observations and conclusions.

Success Stories in ACA Implementation

I define successes as ACA provisions that were implemented substantially as formulated in the statute and that have shown demonstrable positive outcomes.

State Health Insurance Exchanges (Title 1, Subtitle D)

Though both Senate- and House-approved versions of health reform legislation in 2009 incorporated the "health insurance exchange" concept to facilitate the purchase of individual health insurance policies, differences were substantial. The House preferred sole federal management of exchanges in all 50 states by the US Department of Health and Human Services (HHS). The Senate, more deferential to states, gave them right of first refusal, with HHS as backup for nonparticipants. The disagreement ended by default after Senate Democrats lost their 60–seat majority in January 2010 and approving the Senate version became the only pathway to pass a health reform statute.

Senate drafters wrongly assumed that most states would want to establish marketplaces to maintain maximum authority over their individual health insurance markets. Mostly Democratic-controlled state governments stepped forward, initially joined by some Republican leaders in conservative states. As ACA implementation became entrenched partisan warfare, conservative activists convinced political leaders in nearly all Republican-controlled states to reject creating marketplaces that might legitimize the law they despised. The ranks of participating Democratic states thinned because of the ACA's 2013 website catastrophe that disabled the HHS and numerous state websites. By 2016, only 13 states fully ran their own exchanges, nearly all in Democrat-dominated states.

In the state-federal health exchange experiment, we have a verdict: hands down, the 13 states win. Almost across the board, states with their own exchanges have achieved higher enrollment rates than their federally reliant peers, along with lower premiums and better consumer education and protection. They have proven more resilient in withstanding Trump administration moves to discourage enrollment. This makes sense: those using the state marketplace model (SBM) have reputations on the line and are committed to success. For example, between 2016 and 2019, SBM states saw an 11.5% increase in young enrollees, while states with federally facilitated marketplaces experienced an 11.3% drop. While Marketplace premiums across the nation spiked from 2016 to 2018 because of market uncertainty, since 2014 states with federally facilitated marketplaces have seen 87% premium growth while SBM states saw 47% growth (NASHP 2019).

With this evidence, it is unsurprising that policy makers in some states (Maine, New Jersey, New Mexico, and Pennsylvania) are now moving to launch their own exchanges; Nevada opened its own in fall 2019. While it is true that overall federal and state exchange enrollment came substantially below Congressional Budget Office (CBO) expectations in 2010, that is a broader ACA policy issue. Had most states established exchanges, numbers of uninsured would have diminished even more.

Medicaid's Modified Adjusted Gross Income Standard (Title 2, Section 2001)

The saying about Medicaid used to be, "If you've seen one state Medicaid program, you've seen one state Medicaid program." This is still true, but less so because of Title 2 and MAGI, the new uniform national income eligibility standard. Since its establishment in 1965, Medicaid varied enormously across states and the District of Columbia. Some states sought to identify and enroll as many eligible families as possible, while others sought to deter enrollment, making it as challenging as possible to enroll and stay. One method to discourage enrollment was to define household income in as restrictive and exclusionary a manner as legally permissible.

Title 2 changed this dynamic by mandating uniform national rules to determine financial eligibility for Medicaid, subsidized coverage in the exchanges, and the Children's Health Insurance Program (CHIP). The ACA sets one definition for household income, especially what counts and what doesn't count toward that standard (e.g., tips and unemployment compensation count as income, while child support and worker's compensation payments do not). MAGI enables families to move to other states and retain eligibility, even when transitioning between Medicaid and exchange coverage because of household income fluctuation, lessening the dynamic called "churn" (Ryan and Artiga 2015). Milligan (2015) refers to MAGI as one of the ACA's "overlooked virtues." While full MAGI implementation has been slow in some states, others have seen dramatic improvement in coverage renewals.

The Physician Payments Sunshine Act and the Open Payments Website (Title 6, Section 6002)

Over decades, evidence has shown that most physicians and other medical care providers receive gifts, honoraria, and other benefits bestowed by drug and medical device companies to influence medical decision making. To discourage this, ACA crafters placed the Physician Payments Sunshine Act into Title 6, requiring medical industries to disclose to the HHS all non-care-related payments to physicians, teaching hospitals, and others. HHS uses this information to populate its Open Payments website, where anyone can search and view disclosures of payments to physicians, teaching hospitals, and others providers, and to make annual reports to Congress (HHS and CMS 2019). Surprisingly, the Sunshine Act passed with support from pharmaceutical, medical device, and other stakeholders—to stem a proliferation of similar state requirements.

Since the 2013 launch of Open Payments, no sign of mass consumer participation is apparent; one study showed that while 65% of surveyed patients had seen a physician who received an industry payment in the past year, only 12% of knew that payment information was available, and only 5% knew whether their doctor received a payment (Pham-Kanter et al. 2017). On the other hand, the nonprofit investigative journalism group ProPublica has created a user-friendly site called Dollars for Docs (projects .propublica.org/docdollars) that uses the data to document, between 2013 and 2018, $12 billion in payments from 2,191 corporations to 1,036,165 medical providers and 1,249 teaching hospitals. The US Department of Justice, the Food and Drug Administration (FDA), and other federal agencies now cross-reference Open Payments reports with prescriber databases to identify violations of antikickback and false claims statutes (Litman 2018). For those seeking transparency, here it is.

New Medicare Payroll Taxes (Title 9, Section 9015)

The twenty-first century, as of 2020, has seen enactment of three major federal health laws: the 2003 Medicare Modernization Act (MMA), 2010

Affordable Care Act (ACA), and 2015 Medicare and CHIP Reauthorization Act (MACRA). While ACA received zero Republican support, MMA and MACRA had bipartisan support. Of note, MMA and MACRA were mostly deficit financed, creating hundreds of billions in new federal debt. The ACA, in contrast, was completely self-financed, mostly through payment cuts to Medicare providers and care delivery efficiencies in Title 3, and new taxes in Title 9. Tax targets included drug, health insurance, and medical device companies (the latter two were repealed in late 2019's budget deal), and most important, high-income households earning above $200,000 for individuals and $250,000 for families via new Medicare payroll taxes on earned and unearned income.

At $210 billion in projected revenue (2010–19), this last item is the ACA's largest single financing source. It is also distinctly progressive, placing the heaviest burden on the most affluent. Though Republicans attempted to repeal all of Title 9 in their 2017 "repeal and replace" efforts, the new payroll taxes were implemented without incident or even much public notice, until Republicans' 2017 repeal campaign. According to the *New York Times*, the tax hike, especially the 3.8% tax on net investment income, had a significant impact in reducing US income inequality during this decade (Norris 2014). The 0.9% tax on earnings raised $10 billion in 2018, while the net investment income tax raised $27 billion, paid only by the top 5% of income earners and especially the top 1% (Tax Policy Center, n.d.).

Failures in ACA Implementation

Any complex statute results in implementation challenges, positive and negative, expected and surprising. Given the ACA's numerous provisions, it is unsurprising that some failed. These are noteworthy among them.

Consumer Operated and Oriented Plan Program (Title 1, Section 1322)

In summer 2009, Sen. Kent Conrad (D-ND) promoted nonprofit health insurance cooperatives as an alternative to the so-called public option and used his perch on the Senate Finance Committee to secure inclusion in the ACA as the Consumer Operated and Oriented Plan Program (CO-OP). While many observers discounted the provision as window dressing, they were surprised when 23 CO-OPs emerged to serve enrollees in 26 states, with $2.4 billion in federal start-up and solvency loans. The Obama administration took a supportive approach, deciding that CO-OPs might inject needed competition into marketplaces.

In the ACA, Congress authorized up to $6 billion in support, rescinding more than $4 billion between 2011 and 2013 and halting new CO-OPs in 2015 (40 applications were pending). Congress responded positively to insurance industry lobbying to prevent use of federal funds for marketing, by limiting CO-OPs' ability to grow in employer markets and by requiring full loan payback within 5 years. Many CO-OPs ran into early fiscal trouble from multiple directions: some badly over- or underestimated enrollments; many were damaged by the ACA's risk adjustment and risk corridor provisions; others suffered from management deficiencies. By the time a scathing Senate oversight report was released in March 2016, only 10 remained (Permanent Subcommittee on Investigations 2016). As of early 2019, only four remain functioning in five states (Norris 2019).

The ACA's aspiration was for CO-OPs in all 50 states—if not a failure, it is at best a D minus. Who is at fault? Fingers point to ineffective oversight by the Obama administration, congressional Republican sabotage, insurance industry undermining, CO-OP management flaws, and ACA design features. It was all five—how much from each is where arguments begin.

The National Health Care Workforce Commission
(Title 5, Section 5101)

While many ACA elements were fought fiercely among congressional Democrats and Republicans, one provision provoked broad support: the establishment of the National Health Care Workforce Commission, the crown jewel of Title 5, the health workforce part of the law. Modeled on the Medicare Payment Advisory Commission, the commission was tasked to collect data, develop analyses, and make recommendations to Congress, the administration, states, counties, municipalities, and the private sector to develop a healthy workforce better able to meet the needs of evolving American society. The US comptroller general was directed to fill the commission by late 2010. On time, he named 15 experts representing the diversity of health workforce concerns.

Major ACA elements received direct appropriations, thus avoiding annual funding battles that can tie Congress in knots and disable any law or program. Such consideration for the commission was considered unnecessary because of its broad support. In 2011, hats in hands, commission supporters, led by newly designated chairperson Dr. Peter Buerhaus (a nursing workforce expert and now professor at Montana State University), went to Congress seeking $3 million in appropriations as requested by the Obama administration to begin work (Buerhaus and Retchin 2013). Without appropriations, commission members were legally prohibited from even convening. Also, 2011 was the year Republicans reclaimed majority control of the US House of Representatives. Buerhaus and Retchin (2013) describe the expressions of sympathy they received from them, but no support, because the commission was a creature of the vilified ObamaCare.

By late 2019, all staggered terms of commission members have long since expired. The Government Accountability Office labels the commission status as "inactive"; others use the term "dormant." Either way is putting it mildly.

Independent Payment Advisory Board, Title 3, Section 3403

During the ACA's legislative process, complaints arose in fall 2009 that the bill lacked meaningful cost controls. Sen. Jay Rockefeller (D-WV) agreed and won inclusion of the IPAB, a new entity to be composed of 15 members who would be summoned to duty whenever Medicare spending growth exceeded statutory targets. The IPAB would be directed to recommend how to lower Medicare's rate of growth to the spending benchmark, though recommendations could not include eligibility or benefit cuts or tax increases, leaving provider payment cuts as the primary available tool. If Congress failed to pass alternative remedies to save at least as much as would the IPAB's recommendations, then those recommendations would take effect with the force of law. What's more, if an IPAB was not appointed, the HHS secretary was directed to act as the board and make statutorily binding Medicare program changes.

Following ACA enactment, health care provider groups began mobilizing to weaken or repeal the IPAB. In the conservative backlash to the ACA, Sarah Palin, the *Wall Street Journal*, and others identified IPAB as the so-called death panel that would decide whether individual Medicare enrollees would receive medically necessary services (Palin 2010). In the intense ACA implementation period through 2014, the Obama administration chose not to nominate anyone for the IPAB. Once Republicans assumed majority control of the Senate in 2015, chances for approval of any IPAB nominee dropped to zero. But the anti-IPAB provider coalition remained worried about the HHS secretary assuming IPAB powers, even though Medicare per-enrollee spending growth throughout the decade had dropped to historically low rates of increase—in no year between 2013 and 2018 did the rate of Medicare spending growth exceed the CBO's 2010 benchmark. Democrats also worried about how the Trump administration might use IPAB's power to make changes to Medicare.

On February 9, 2018, the US House and Senate voted to repeal IPAB in the Bipartisan Budget Act of 2018, signed that day by President Trump. In its analysis of the enacted ACA, the CBO estimated that IPAB would save the federal government $15.5 billion through 2019. Actual savings from lower than projected inflation were far greater than that amount. IPAB's demise is another indication of the difficulty in implementing and sustaining health care cost control mechanisms—even those that can survive the legislative process.

Community Living Assistance Services and Supports (Title 8)

CLASS was a personal priority for my former boss, the late Sen. Edward Kennedy (D-MA), who avidly sought a way to provide cash support to temporarily or permanently disabled Americans to assist them in living independently outside institutions. Because the ACA already included a mandate on individuals to purchase health insurance (in Title 1), congressional leaders deemed the inclusion of a second mandate for CLASS as politically infeasible. CLASS became Title 8 of the ACA, structured as a voluntary insurance program in which anyone could enroll and receive benefits after 5 years of uninterrupted premium payments. Because of its voluntary design, it also faced massive risk selection problems, among others. After Kennedy's death, his close friend Sen. Chris Dodd (D-CT) secured its inclusion despite opposition from most Republicans and influential Democrats, such as Senate Finance Chair Max Baucus (D-MT).

In October 2011, the Obama administration declared CLASS to be unworkable, with HHS Secretary Kathleen Sebelius declaring: "I do not see a viable path forward for CLASS implementation at this time" (Wayne and Armstrong 2011). CLASS repeal was signed by President Obama on January 1, 2013—the only ACA title to be repealed in toto. In the bill, Congress established a special commission to consider alternatives—a commission that proved unable to agree on any alternative.

Connie Garner, a neonatal intensive care nurse practitioner, was Senator Kennedy's point person on CLASS, its fiercest advocate. Garner now runs Allies for Independence, a national advocacy organization that continues advocating for the cause. Perhaps most significant, in May 2019 Washington Governor Jay Inslee signed into law the nation's first public and state-operated long-term care insurance program that is scheduled to begin in 2022, to be financed by a mandatory new tax of $0.58 on every $100 of income, going into a state trust fund (Lieber 2019).

Mixed Results in ACA Implementation

Calorie Labeling for Chain Restaurant Menus (Title 4, Section 4205)

In the first decade of the twenty-first century, in response to the rapidly growing obesity epidemic among Americans of all ages, some local governments began requiring chain restaurants to post the number of calories for each food item on their menus and menu boards. Initially resistant, the restaurant industry found it was unable to block passage of local laws that varied substantially in details. To avoid a regulatory Tower of Babel, the industry endorsed a national calorie posting requirement in Title 4, the public health part of the law. Though scheduled to start in 2013, the FDA encountered intense conflict over regulatory details from movie theaters, pizza chains, grocery stores, and others that nearly derailed the entire system until May 2018, when it was finally implemented by the Trump administration.

Many food chains did not wait until 2018 to begin posting, thus enabling early research on the practice. Two findings dominate the literature. First, initial posting of calorie content triggers at best a short-lived reduction in consumed calories (Long et al. 2015). A Cochrane review estimated as much as a 50–calorie impact per meal, though it considered the quality of that evidence "low" (Crockett et al. 2018). Second, in response to calorie labeling, behavior change is observable and sustained by numerous restaurants chains that have trended toward discontinuing high-calorie items, thus reducing calorie content without relying on individual behavior change (Bleich, Wolfson, and Jarlenski 2017; Bleich et al. 2018). Though judgments on its effectiveness vary, the law seems here to stay.

Elder Justice Act (Title 6, Subtitle H)

A 2010 study concluded that 11% of individuals age 60 and over reported receiving abusive behavior in the previous year, including verbal, financial, or physical mistreatment by family members or others, a number experts regard as an underestimate (Acierno et al. 2010). Former Sen. John Breaux (D-LA) first filed the Elder Justice Act in 2002 to initiate a coordinated and comprehensive approach to elder abuse and to advance state-level responses. After Breaux's retirement, Sen. Richard Durbin (D-IL) and former Sen. Orrin Hatch (R-UT) picked up the cause. After years of trying, the national Elder Justice Coalition saw their proposal become part of Title 6. For elder justice advocates, it was a historic landmark.

Developments since enactment have been disappointing. In 2017, the Congressional Research Service issued a status report on the act (Colello 2017). On the positive side, a HHS Elder Justice Coordinating Council was established in 2012 with representation from the US Department of Justice and HHS. Conversely, Congress appropriated none of the authorized funding for elder abuse forensic centers, none for enhancement of abuse prevention in long-term care facilities, none for grants to support adult protective services, and none for the Long-Term Care Ombudsman grants/training program or for a national nurse aide registry.

In fiscal years 2012 and 2013, the Obama administration diverted $8 million from the ACA's Public Health and Prevention Fund for Adult Protective Services. In 2015 and 2016, the first time since enactment, Congress appropriated $4 and $8 million, respectively, for similar activities—after the ACA's funding authorization expired. Though marginal advances have been achieved since 2010, the great promises of the Elder Justice Act have not materialized. State governments and advocates continue fighting the epidemic without a full-on federal partner.

Biologics Price Competition and Innovation Act (Title 7)

Few ACA issues instigated more intense stakeholder conflict and hardball lobbying than Title 7 directing the FDA to create a regulatory pathway to license biological products shown to be "biosimilar" or interchangeable with a licensed biopharmaceutical drug. The doorway opened in 2014, and as of November 2019, the FDA has approved 25 biosimilar products.

The model for Title 7 was the 1984 Hatch Waxman Act that unleashed the generic drug revolution in the US pharmaceutical sector—today nearly 90% of prescribed drugs in the United States are generics selling at a fraction of brand-name prices. The generic model is imperfect because the process to make biosimilars, containing live viruses, is distinctly different from commodity manufacturing of traditional generics. Those hoping for many biosimilar products and dramatically lower prices were engaged in wishful thinking.

While every stakeholder—drug and biotechnology companies, business, labor, consumers, insurers—wanted to create the biosimilar pathway, drug and biotech companies wanted extended patent protection for no less than 12 years, while other stakeholders wanted no more than 5 years. Pharma/biotech won 12 years, another factor that has slowed the market.

While the CBO estimated a mere $7 billion in federal budget savings between 2010 and 2019, a recent RAND study projects $54 billion (with a range of $24–150 billion) between 2017 and 2026 (Mulcahy, Hlavka, and Case 2018). While many are dissatisfied with the market impact of biosimilars, ACA authors always assumed this would be a robust market for the 2020s and beyond.

Conclusion

The ACA includes an extensive collection of health policies, some newly developed between 2009 and 2010 and others that had waited years for a window of opportunity. The law is judged mostly on its top-line policies relating to access, insurance, cost control, and delivery system reform. The overall collection of ACA policies is far more diverse and extensive than recognized, far more than the 11 assessed in this review. Some have succeeded while others failed, and others are still works in progress. Many, perhaps most, of these policies would never have seen the light of day were it not for the generational opportunity provided by the ACA process. Many of these lesser-known policies continue making a meaningful impact, for better or worse, within the US health care system. Like nearly everything else involving the ACA, judgments usually vary depending on one's ideological views toward the base law.

The legendary Russian actor and director Konstantin Stanislavski is reported to have claimed, "There are no small parts, only small actors." We can notice, 10 years later, that in all of the ACA's secondary roles, smaller and yet fully attentive publics pay close attention. For affected stakeholders, these bit parts have an ongoing, meaningful, and unrecognized impact on America's health care system.

▪ ▪ ▪

John E. McDonough is professor of practice at the Harvard T. H. Chan School of Public Health. Between 2008 and 2010 he served as a senior advisor on national health reform to the US Senate Committee on Health, Education, Labor, and Pensions, where he worked on the Affordable Care Act. Between 2003 and 2008 he was executive director of Health Care for All, a Massachusetts consumer health advocacy organization, where he played a leading role in the passage of the 2006 Massachusetts Health Reform Law. From 1985 to 1997 he was a member of the Massachusetts House of Representatives.
jmcdonough@hsph.harvard.edu

Acknowledgments

Special thanks to Karen Jiang for research assistance.

References

Acierno, Ron, Melba A. Hernandez, Ananda B. Amstadter, Heidi S. Resnick, Kenneth Steve, Wendy Muzzy, and Dean G. Kilpatrick. 2010. "Prevalence and Correlates of Emotional, Physical, Sexual, and Financial Abuse and Potential Neglect in the United States: The National Elder Mistreatment Study." *American Journal of Public Health* 100, no. 2: 292–97. doi.org/10.2105/AJPH.2009.163089.

Bleich, Sara N., Julia A. Wolfson, and Marian P. Jarlenski. 2017. "Calorie Changes in Large Chain Restaurants." *American Journal of Preventive Medicine* 50, no. 1: e1–e8. doi.org/10.1016/j.amepre.2015.05.007.

Bleich, Sara N., Alyssa J. Moran, Marian P. Jarlenski, and Julia A. Wolfson. 2018. "Higher-Calorie Menu Items Eliminated in Large Chain Restaurants." *American Journal of Preventive Medicine* 54, no. 2: 214–20. doi.org/10.1016/j.amepre.2017.11.004.

Buerhaus, Peter I., and Sheldon M. Retchin. 2013. "The Dormant National Health Care Workforce Commission Needs Congressional Funding to Fulfill Its Promise." *Health Affairs* 32, no. 11: 2021–24. doi.org/10.1377/hlthaff.2013.0385.

Colello, Kirsten J. 2017. "The Elder Justice Act: Background and Issues for Congress." Congressional Research Service, January 24. fas.org/sgp/crs/misc/R43707.pdf.

Crockett, Rachel A., Sarah E. King, Theresa M. Marteau, A. T. Prevost, Giacomo Bignardi, Nia W. Roberts, Brendon Stubbs, Gareth J. Hollands, and Susan A. Jebb. 2018. "Nutritional Labelling for Healthier Food." *Cochrane Database of Systematic Reviews* 2018, no. 2, art. no. CD009315. doi.org/10.1002/14651858.CD009315.pub2.

HHS (US Department of Health and Human Services) and CMS (Centers for Medicare and Medicaid Services). 2019. "Annual Report to Congress on the Open Payments Program." April. www.cms.gov/OpenPayments/Downloads/report-to-congress.pdf.

Lieber, Ron. 2019. "New Tax Will Help Washington Residents Pay for Long-Term Care." *New York Times*, May 13. www.nytimes.com/2019/05/13/business/washington-long-term-care.html.

Long, Michael W., Deirdre K. Tobias, Angie L. Cradock, Holly Batchelder, and Steven L. Gortmaker. 2015. "Systematic Review and Meta-Analysis of the Impact of Restaurant Menu Calorie Labeling." *American Journal of Public Health* 105, no. 5: e11–e24. doi.org/10.2105/AJPH.2015.302570.

Milligan, Charles. 2015. "From Coverage to Care: Addressing the Issue of Churn." *Journal of Health Politics, Policy and Law* 40, no. 1: 227–32. doi.org/10.1215/03616878-2854829.

Mulcahy, Andrew W., Jakub P. Hlavka, and Spencer R. Case. 2018. "Biosimilar Cost Savings in the United States." *RAND Health Quarterly* 7, no. 4: 3. www.rand.org /pubs/periodicals/health-quarterly/issues/v7/n4/03.html.

NASHP (National Academy for State Health Policy). 2019. "State Based Health Insurance Marketplace Performance." September. nashp.org/wp-content/uploads /2019/09/SBM-slides-final_SeptMtgs-9_23_2019.pdf.

Norris, Floyd. 2014. "Merely Rich and Superrich: The Tax Gap Is Narrowing." *New York Times*, April 18. www.nytimes.com/2014/04/18/business/merely-rich-and -superrich-the-tax-gap-is-narrowing.html.

Norris, Louise. 2019. "CO-OP Health Plans: Patients' Interests First." Health insurance.org, January 3. www.healthinsurance.org/obamacare/co-op-health-plans -put-patients-interests-first/.

Palin, Sarah. 2010. "Why I Support the Ryan Roadmap." *Wall Street Journal*, December 10. www.wsj.com/articles/SB10001424052748703766704576009322 838245628.

Pham-Kanter, Genevieve, Michelle M. Mello, Lisa Soleymani Lehmann, Eric G. Campbell, and Daniel Carpenter. 2017. "Public Awareness of and Contact with Physicians Who Receive Industry Payments: A National Survey." *Journal of General Internal Medicine* 32, no. 7: 767–74. doi.org/10.1007/s11606-017-4012-3.

Ryan, Jennifer, and Samantha Artiga. 2015. "Renewals in Medicaid and CHIP." Kaiser Family Foundation, June 26. harbageconsulting.com/wp-content/uploads/2016/09 /Renewals-in-Medicaid-and-CHIP-Implementation-of-Streamlined-ACA-Policies -and-the-Potential-Role-of-Managed-Care-Plans.pdf.

Tax Policy Center. n.d. *Briefing Book: What Tax Changes Did the Affordable Care Act Make?* www.taxpolicycenter.org/briefing-book/what-tax-changes-did-affordable -care-act-make (accessed February 10, 2020).

US Senate Permanent Subcommittee on Investigations. 2016. "Failure of the Affordable Care Act Health Insurance CO-OPs." March 10. www.hsgac.senate.gov /imo/media/doc/Majority%20Staff%20Report%20–%20Failure%20of%20the%20 Affordable%20Care%20Act%20Health%20Insurance%20CO-OPs.pdf.

Wayne, Alex, and Drew Armstrong. 2011. "Kennedy-Backed Long-Term Care Program Scrapped by Sebelius." Bloomberg, October 14. www.bloomberg.com/news /articles/2011-10-14/u-s-won-t-start-class-long-term-care-insurance-sebelius-says.

Race, Politics, and the Affordable Care Act

Jamila Michener
Cornell University

Abstract   The political processes surrounding the Affordable Care Act (ACA) offer valuable lessons about race and politics in the United States. In particular, the ACA underscores a critical tension between politics and policy in a racialized polity: even when policies are intended to target and address racial disparities, politics can undermine the steps necessary to do so. Close scrutiny of the ACA during its first decade reveals how race intersects with politics to render public policy less equitable and more vulnerable to erosion. Ultimately, this analysis points to the ways that racialized political processes are formidable barriers to equitable material outcomes. By examining such processes and making them visible, this article elucidates the possibilities, limits, and contours of public policy as a mechanism for achieving racial justice.

Keywords   Affordable Care Act, race, politics

Analyzing the political processes surrounding the Affordable Care Act (ACA) can teach us valuable lessons about race and politics in the United States. In particular, the ACA underscores a critical tension between politics and policy in a racialized polity:[1] even when policies are intended to winnow racial disparities, politics can undermine the steps necessary to do so. Close attention to the implementation of the ACA reveals how race intersects with politics to render public policy less equitable. Only by

---

1. Following Gotham (2000) and Bonilla Silva (1997), I define racialization as economic, social, and political processes by which "people are sorted into racial categories, resources are distributed along racial lines, and state policy shapes and is shaped by the racial contours of society" (Gotham 2000: 293).

Journal of Health Politics, Policy and Law, Vol. 45, No. 4, August 2020
DOI 10.1215/03616878-8255481   © 2020 by Duke University Press

scrutinizing such processes can we discern how policies and politics might be wielded to achieve racial justice in health care.

The ACA and Racial Inequality

The ACA was designed to reduce health inequities based on race and ethnicity (Ossei-Owusu 2016). The text of the original bill (Pub. L. No. 111–148. 3–23–2010) contained 34 references to "disparities," 28 references to either "discrimination" or "non-discrimination," 33 instances using either the word *racial* or *race*, and 35 instances using either the word *ethnicity* or *ethnic*. Though Barack Obama's approach to advancing his policy goals was often deracialized, the explicit emphasis on race in the ACA reveals a pronounced goal of diminishing racial disparities (Gillion 2016; Lewis, Dowe, and Franklin 2013). Such intentions notwithstanding, the ACA reflects an incongruity between politics and policy. On the one hand, health care politics became more deeply racialized during the presidency of Barack Obama and has remained so (Banks 2014; Fiscella 2016; Knowles, Lowery, and Schaumberg 2010; Maxwell and Shields 2014; McCabe 2019; Mitchell and Dowe 2019; Morone 2018; Tesler 2012). On the other hand, ACA policy was a harbinger of racial promise. Even in the face of antagonistic racial politics, with white Americans disproportionately opposing Obamacare, the policies of the ACA had "the potential to truly alter the landscape of racial and ethnic health disparities in the United States" (Mitchell 2015: e-66). Indeed, from the vantage point of those concerned with the legacy of racism in the United States, the ACA was viewed as "a stealthy civil-rights achievement of the Obama presidency, promising to make health care less of a financial burden, end disparities in health-care coverage, ease barriers to access for people of color, and subsidize preventative health-care services that proved especially lacking in black neighborhoods" (Newkirk 2016).

In retrospect, some of these expectations proved true. The ACA reduced racial/ethnic disparities in health insurance coverage, access to care, and health care utilization (Buchmueller et al. 2016; Chaudry, Jackson, and Glied 2019; Chen at al. 2016; Gutierrez 2018; Lipton, Decker, and Sommers 2019; McMorrow et al. 2016; Park et al. 2018). The reduction of insurance coverage gaps was one of the most salient ways that the ACA had a salutary effect on racial inequity. Between 2013 and 2017, the coverage gap between black and white Americans declined from 11.0 to 5.3 percentage points (Chaudry, Jackson, and Glied 2019). Similarly, during the same period, the coverage gap between Hispanics and non-Hispanic whites dropped from 25.4 to 16.6 percentage points.

Despite such good news, the story of race and the ACA is not a straightforward narrative of success. Racial imbalances in health care access and quality persist in the post-ACA era (Artiga, Orgera, and Damico 2019; Buchmueller et al. 2016; Yue, Rasmussen, and Ponce 2018). Moreover, the progress of the ACA in lessening racial disparities has begun to plateau or reverse (Artiga, Orgera, and Damico 2019). Insurance coverage is again a good example. After the above-mentioned improvements in coverage rates between 2013 and 2017, the overall uninsured rate rose from 7.9% in 2017 to 8.5% in 2018 (Berchick, Barnett, and Upton 2019). Hispanic Americans were most affected, with a 1.6–percentage-point increase in their uninsured rate.

To better understand this and other shortcomings of the ACA with respect to racial equity, we must look to politics. Doing so uncovers distinctive patterns that have stunted the ACA's ability to properly function as a "civil rights achievement." In this vein, I make two observations. First, even the most salient inequality-reducing feature of the ACA—Medicaid expansion—has endured politically induced variation, attenuating its effectiveness in diminishing racial disparities. Second, beyond Medicaid expansion, many of the numerous features of the ACA that explicitly target racial disparities have proven unstable or limited because their implementation has been contingent on political conditions.

The common thread uniting both of these points is that racialized politics constrains American public policy as a tool for equity. To detail this claim more precisely, I delineate complex and consequential connections between race, policy, and politics in American health care.

The Racialized Politics of Medicaid Expansion

As it was originally designed, one of the ACA's boldest and most promising mechanisms for reducing racial inequities was the expansion of Medicaid. Per the initial formulation of the ACA, Medicaid expansion would have offered public health insurance to all Americans with incomes at or below 138% of the federal poverty line. To secure the participation of every state, the federal government brandished both a carrot and a stick. The carrot consisted of generous federal funding that would cover 100% of the costs of expansion for nearly 3 years (from the beginning of 2014 through the end of 2016) and then gradually phase down to 90% by 2020. The stick meant that states refusing expansion would forfeit all of their federal Medicaid funding (not just the extra expansion resources). This combination of incentives and sanctions was intended to ensure the geographic consistency of Medicaid expansion, an outcome that would have been a major departure from the norm. Prior to the enactment of the ACA, access to Medicaid was limited and highly unequal (Michener 2018). Variable categorical eligibility criteria at both the national and state levels meant that program benefits were heterogeneous across groups (with children, the elderly, pregnant women, and other specific groups often receiving more generous benefits) and across states (with some locales offering a wider scope of benefits and broader eligibility criteria than others). If Medicaid expansion had proceeded as originally planned, this patchwork policy design would have been augmented with a more standardized national approach applied to all Americans at or below 138% of the federal poverty line. Though the planned expansionary tack was not explicitly race based, the outsized presence of blacks and Latinos among the population of Americans living in or near poverty (e.g., 20% of Medicaid beneficiaries are black and 30% are Latino; KFF n.d.) meant that uniform national expansion of Medicaid would have had inequality-reducing racial effects.

Despite the initial objectives of the ACA, political processes fundamentally altered its course. Just over 2 years after the passage of the law (and before its full implementation), the Supreme Court issued a decision declaring Medicaid expansion partially unconstitutional. In *National Federation of Independent Business v. Sebelius*, 567 U.S. 519 (2012), the court held that by threatening noncompliant states with the loss of all Medicaid funds, the 2010 expansion was coercive. The *Sebelius* decision transformed the trajectory of the ACA, empowering states to eschew the expansion if they saw fit to do so. Many states did. Decisions about whether to expand largely (though not entirely) fell along partisan lines (Barrilleaux and Rainey 2014; Callaghan and Jacobs 2016; Jacobs and Callaghan 2013). States with Democratic legislative majorities and Democratic executives adopted the expansion most swiftly, while states with divided governments or Republican legislative majorities were less likely to do so, particularly in the South.

The intercession of the Supreme Court in the *Sebelius* case was consistent with the enduring role of federalism in the American political system, specifically with regard to health care, and especially concerning racialized resources (Michener 2018). People of color have long been disproportionately disadvantaged by federalism (Brown 2003; Lieberman and Lapinski 2001; Lowndes, Novkov, and Warren 2008; Miller 2008; Riker 1964; Soss, Fording, and Schram 2011; Tani 2016). Indeed, federalism "has been one of the chief bulwarks of racial domination in the United States" (Brown 2003: 56). Particularly (but not exclusively) with respect to health care policies, racial disparities have been the frequent outcome of enhancing state discretion (Michener 2018). Given this larger national historical context, the court's decision in *Sebelius* had clear negative implications for the racial equitability of health resources.

The most concrete upshot of *Sebelius* is that many southern states have been able to evade Medicaid expansion (see fig. 1). The resulting racial distributional patterns have been stark. A 2015 Kaiser Family Foundation report (Artiga, Damico, and Garfield 2015) found that more than 60% of uninsured poor black adults excluded from Medicaid due to states' refusal to expand (i.e. those in the coverage gap) lived in just four southern states: Georgia (19%), Texas (16%), Florida (14%), and Louisiana (11%). Among Latinos, the patterns were even more striking. Nearly 8 in 10 Latinos in the coverage gap resided in just two states: Texas (52%) and Florida (27%). More generally, many of the southern states that declined to adopt were places with large shares of blacks (Mississippi, 38%; Louisiana, 32%; Georgia, 31%; Alabama, 27%; South Carolina, 27%) or Latinos (Texas, 40%; Florida, 26%). Ultimately, the racial demographics of the South have meant that the concentration of nonexpansion states in the region is a source of significant racial inequality in health care access.

Crucially, this inequity was induced by racialized political decisions. Numerous studies have demonstrated this. Lanford and Quadagno (2015) found that racial resentment was closely linked to Medicaid expansion, with lower racial sympathy and higher racial resentment (on the state level) correlated with stronger resistance to Medicaid expansion. Grogan and Park (2017) found that Medicaid expansion was racialized in terms of public support (with whites much less likely to support expansion) and policy adoption (with state expansion decisions positively correlated with white opinion but uncorrelated with nonwhite support). Grogan and Park also found that when the size of the black population increased and white support was relatively low, states were significantly less likely to expand Medicaid. This helps us to make sense of nonexpansion in southern states with significant health care needs but large black populations. Racial representational disparities combined with racial differences in policy preferences have been barriers to Medicaid expansion. As a result, there are significantly higher proportions of uninsured Americans in nonexpansion states, with the largest and most evident disadvantages among people of color (see fig. 2).

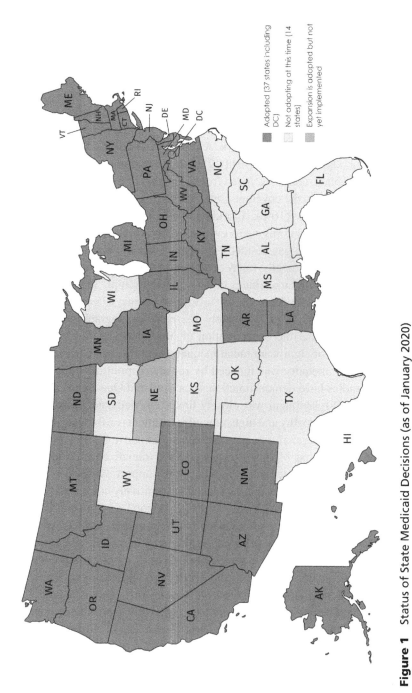

Figure 1 Status of State Medicaid Decisions (as of January 2020)

Source: Map created using mapchart.net under CC BY-SA 4.0.

Legend:
Adopted (37 states including DC)
Not adopting at this time (14 states)
Expansion is adopted but not yet implemented

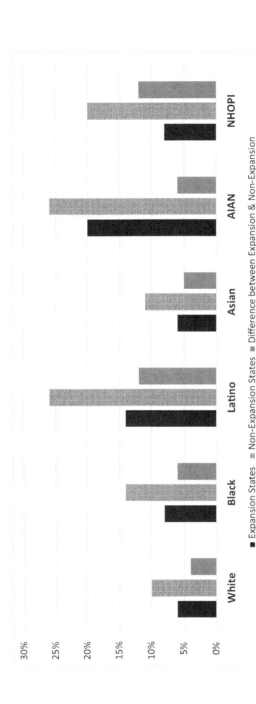

Figure 2 Uninsured Rate among Nonelderly by Race/Ethnicity and State Medicaid Expansion Status

Notes: NHOPI=Native Hawaiians and Other Pacific Islanders; AIAN=American Indians and Alaska Natives. All values reflect the statistically significant difference between expansion and nonexpansion states at the p < 0.05 level.

Source: Kaiser Family Foundation analysis of the 2017 American Community Survey.

The Racialized Politics of Medicaid Demonstration Waivers

State Medicaid demonstration (section 1115) waivers are also crucial elements of the ACA with implications for race and politics. Waivers provide states with the flexibility to implement new policies that (ostensibly) benefit state residents. In the post-ACA era, waivers have offered states an avenue for shaping Medicaid to suit their political prerogatives. In particular, section 1115 waivers have allowed Republicans who may otherwise be loath to adopt Medicaid expansion to do so, thus providing insurance to thousands of low-income state residents while signaling a distance from the Democrats who passed the ACA. The unprecedented uses of 1115 waivers in the post-ACA period are racialized as a result of racial disproportionalities in Medicaid, broader economic and social inequities, and racial biases at the root of policies such as work requirements.

Arkansas is a prime illustration. In March 2018 the state proposed the Arkansas Works program via an amendment to a prior section 1115 waiver. The previous waiver (2013) had already placed Arkansas at the vanguard of innovation through a Medicaid demonstration that created what came to be known as the "private option."[2] By initiating Arkansas Works, the 2018 amendment to the initial waiver went in a very different direction, heavily focusing on work-reporting requirements. The Centers for Medicare and Medicaid Services approved the proposal, ushering in a key change: a "work and community engagement" requirement for members of the expansion group under age 50. This necessitated that during any given month beneficiaries must either meet an exemption (e.g., medially frail, pregnant, etc.) or complete 80 hours of qualifying activities, including employment, education, and community service.

The most prominent result of this policy was massive coverage loss. In just 7 months more than 18,000 people were disenrolled (Wagner and Schubel 2019). Early research surveying low-income Arkansans has confirmed that work-reporting requirements are associated with a substantial loss of Medicaid coverage, a rise in the percentage of uninsured persons, and no significant changes in employment (Sommers et al. 2019). Most germane, the case of Arkansas epitomizes the significance of race in

2. Arkansas's initial 2013 Medicaid expansion (under Democratic governor Mike Beebe) occurred through a 1115 waiver that allowed the use of state Medicaid funds to provide premium assistance to eligible beneficiaries, enabling them to purchase private health insurance via the state health insurance marketplace. This allowed Arkansas to insure roughly 220,000 Medicaid beneficiaries via commercial provider networks.

understanding Medicaid waivers. Racial disproportionalities in the state's Medicaid program mean that black Americans are particularly vulnerable to the negative effects of Arkansas Works (Michener 2019; Sommers et al. 2019). Though black people account for less than 13% of the US population and only 15% of Arkansas residents, they make up 26% of Medicaid beneficiaries in the state. This means that 47% of black Arkansans rely on Medicaid (compared to 25% of white Arkansans and 31% of Latino Arkansans). Any policy that results in the large-scale loss of Medicaid coverage is likely to have lopsided racial consequences. Indeed, consistent with this expectation, recent analyses of the effects of work requirements in the Supplemental Nutrition Assistance Program and Temporary Assistance to Needy Families show that for both programs black Americans were unevenly affected by work requirements (Brantley, Pillai, and Ku 2019; Hall and Burrowes 2019). These studies suggest that, even beyond Arkansas, work requirements do not bode well for racial equity.[3]

Over and above racial disproportionalities in Medicaid, broader social and economic racial biases also shape the effects of work requirements. For example, research demonstrates how detrimental a criminal record is to labor market outcomes, especially for black people (Pager 2008). In a state like Arkansas, the incarceration rate for blacks is very high relative to whites, making a criminal record a barrier to employment for significant subsets of black Arkansans (see fig. 3). By necessitating employment as a qualification for receiving Medicaid, work requirements can thus intersect with disparities in other institutional venues (labor market, criminal justice system) to spread disadvantage across arenas.

Even beyond the disadvantage of a criminal record, compelling evidence points to wide-ranging racial discrimination in low-wage labor markets (Bertrand and Mullainathan 2004; Pager, Bonikowski, and Western 2009). The black unemployment rate is regularly twice that of white unemployment (Wilson 2019). Conditioning Medicaid benefits on seeking and finding work is more burdensome to racially marginalized populations facing significant structural obstacles to employment.

Race is also an imperative aspect of the politics of Medicaid demonstration waivers because the assumptions buoying support for policies like work requirements are themselves racialized. Many Americans

3. Medicaid work requirements have been approved in ten states: Arizona, Arkansas, Indiana, Kentucky, Michigan, New Hampshire, Ohio, Utah, South Carolina, and Wisconsin. In four of these, work requirements have been set aside by state courts (Kentucky, Arkansas, Michigan, and New Hampshire). In several others, they have not yet been implemented (Arizona, Wisconsin, Utah, and Ohio). Numerous other states have pending waivers that await approval, including several states with substantial black populations (Mississippi, Georgia, and Tennessee).

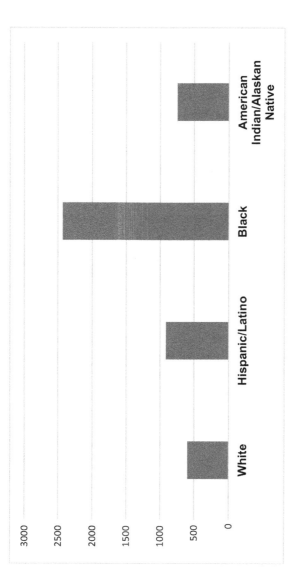

Figure 3 Arkansas Incarceration Rates by Race/Ethnicity

Source: Prison Policy Initiative.

overestimate the presence of black people on welfare rolls (Delaney and Edwards-Levy 2018). Racial stereotypes about undeserving black people taking advantage of government largesse underlie widespread opposition to public benefits, motivating support for policies that make those benefits harder to get (Brown-Iannuzzi et al. 2019; Gilens 1999).

Race and the ACA: Beyond Expansion

Many ACA provisions directly targeted racial disparities. These policies cover a gamut of issues, but their overarching goal is to explicitly marshal the resources of the federal government to reduce health disparities. Three illustrative initiatives in the ACA include:

1. Consistent and systematized health data collection by race, ethnicity, and language
2. Increased racial and ethnic diversity in the health care workforce
3. Nondiscrimination in health programs and activities

All three policy emphases reflect potential mechanisms for advancing health equity (Andrulis et al. 2013; Bristow, Butler, and Smedley, 2004; Dovidio and Fiske 2012; Ulmer, McFadden, and Nerenz 2009).

As some of the ACA's most targeted efforts to confront racial inequality, the implementation and politics of these policies are instructive. Table 1 summarizes some specific statutes, identifies the entities responsible for implementing them, and details the funding associated with each.[4] The key takeaway is that implementation is highly contingent on political conditions (e.g., the positioning of federal bureaucrats, and recurring appropriations). Given this reality, ACA statutes directly confronting race (those with the most overt "civil rights" implications) have been acutely vulnerable to "inconsistent and fluctuating levels of federal engagement" (King 2017: 357). This has been especially true in the hyperpolarized partisan political environment that shapes ACA implementation (Béland, Rocco, and Waddan 2015). The consequence has been "the slowing down or outright death of federal civil rights activism" because the "enforcement of policy is weak. Many of the institutional reforms and national standards needed for amelioration are often given insufficient resources for effective implementation" (King 2017: 357–58). A closer look at the trajectory of the data collection, workforce diversification, and nondiscrimination initiatives underscores this.

---

4. Table 1 does not provide an exhaustive accounting of all relevant provisions. The ACA contains a vast array of policies, and even those highlighted here are more detailed and nuanced than there is space to elaborate.

Table 1 Policy Design of Key Race-Specific ACA Provisions

Policy	Issue	Section	Implementation	Funding
Require population surveys to collect data on race, ethnicity, and language	Data collection	4302	Office of the National Coordinator for Health Information Technology	As necessary
Collect disparities data in Medicaid and CHIP	Data collection	4302	Health and Human Services (HHS) Secretary	As necessary
Monitor health disparities in federally funded programs	Data collection	4302	HHS Secretary	As necessary
Increase diversity among primary care providers	Workforce diversity	5301	HHS Secretary	$125 million (2010)
Increase diversity among long-term care providers	Workforce diversity	5302	HHS Secretary	$10 million (2011–13)
Increase diversity among dentists	Workforce diversity	5303	HHS Secretary	$30 million (2010)
Increase diversity among mental health providers	Workforce diversity	5306	HHS Secretary	$25 million (2010–13)
Increase diversity in nursing professions	Workforce diversity	5309	HHS Secretary	$35,500 per student (2010–11)
Support for low-income health profession/home care aid training	Workforce diversity	5507	HHS and Department of Labor	$85 million (2010–18)
Nondiscrimination in federal health programs and exchanges	Discrimination	1557	HHS Secretary	Unspecified

Source: Affordable Care Act; Andrulis et al. 2010

Race/Ethnicity Data Collection

Section 4302(a) of the ACA stipulates that the Department of Health and Humans Services (HHS) secretary "shall ensure that, by not later than 2 years after the date of enactment of this title, any federally conducted or supported health care or public health program, activity or survey (including Current Population Surveys and American Community Surveys conducted by the Bureau of Labor Statistics and the Bureau of the Census) collects and reports, to the extent practicable—(A) data on race, ethnicity, sex, primary language, and disability status for applicants, recipients, or participants." The objective of this statute was to "support a more focused national strategy to eliminate health and health care disparities among Medicaid and CHIP enrollees" (Burwell 2014: 2).

Particularly crucial is that the main implementing authority is the HHS secretary—a salient and high-profile political appointee. Between 2010 and 2016, when HHS was run by appointees of President Barack Obama, there was significant federal activity related to enforcing section 4302. The *Federal Register* recorded 15 rules that cited section 4302, most between 2012 and 2016 (National Archives n.d.). In the 3–year period following that (between the time the Trump administration took control of HHS in January 2017 and early January 2020) only three rules have cited section 4302. While race/ethnicity data have "remained largely incomplete," there is little indication that data collection remains a federal priority (Ng et al. 2017). Near exclusive reliance on the HHS, a politically salient bureaucracy run by a political appointee, has limited the effectiveness of section 4302.

Workforce Diversity

The ACA contains numerous provisions to enhance racial diversity within the American health care workforce. Many have proven difficult to implement. Even during the Obama administration, a polarized Congress refused to appropriate $3 million to establish the National Health Care Workforce Commission as stipulated by ACA section 5101. Securing appropriations for other aspects of the law related to workforce diversity has been similarly challenging. Statutes related to workforce diversity remain either unfunded or underfunded.[5] Such programs are supported "in

---

5. One important exception worth studying further is the Health Profession Opportunity Grant, authorized via section 5507 of the ACA. This grant project has received consistent funding from Congress.

intent" by the ACA but have perennially faced severe resource constraints (Andrulis et al. 2013). The shift in federal priorities since the election of President Trump has further imperiled funding. The fiscal year 2020 budget proposal for HHS proposed eliminating $88 million for diversity training and $151 million for nursing workforce development (DHHS n.d.). Given continued partisan polarization, it is not at all clear "whether the resources and political will to support a broad spectrum of critical programs and actions will be sufficient to meet service goals and people's need" (Andrulis et al. 2013).

Nondiscrimination

Section 1557, the nondiscrimination provision of the ACA, prohibits discrimination in health care programs on the basis of race. Building on existing federal civil rights laws, section 1557 extends nondiscrimination protections to individuals participating in "any health program or activity, any part of which is receiving Federal financial assistance." Though 1557 did not mandate follow-up regulatory activity, the Obama administration reinforced the law by proposing a "final rule" for implementation (81 C.F.R. 31375). Among other things, the final rule required that covered entities post notices of nondiscrimination in the top 15 languages spoken statewide. These requirements were most directly relevant to people with limited English proficiency, a population that is 88% nonwhite (Batalova and Zong 2016).

Section 1557 has been directly undermined by shifting political winds. In May 2019, the Office for Civil Rights and HHS proposed to revise the final rule issued by the Obama administration in 2016 (National Archives 2019). The 2019 iteration of the rule repealed requirements "to mail beneficiaries, enrollees, and others, notices concerning non-discrimination and the availability of language assistance services." To justify this change, the Office for Civil Right and HHS point to Executive Order 13765, "Minimizing the Economic Burden of the Patient Protection and Affordable Care Act Pending Repeal" (2017). This order asserts the federal government's goal of curtailing the financial burdens of the ACA and directs executive branch agency heads in charge of ACA enforcement to "exercise all authority and discretion available to them to waive, defer, grant exemptions from, or delay the implementation of any provision or requirement of the Act that would impose a fiscal burden."

There is not yet any accounting of the precise effects of such regulatory change on racial health disparities. The larger point, however, is that the politics of the ACA regulatory process unraveled antidiscrimination policies that many people saw as a step forward for racial equity. Indeed, HHS received nearly 156,000 comments responding to its 2019 regulatory change. A (unsystematic) review of these comments indicates that many of them were in opposition to the rule. Yet, the scope that the ACA left for regulatory and bureaucratic maneuvering enabled important policies to be tightly tethered to political conditions.

Conclusion

In a polity where race is a political flashpoint, ACA policies meant to (indirectly or directly) address racial disparities were politically significant steps. Yet, those steps were deeply precarious. In this way, the ACA epitomizes a difficult problem in American politics: the distance between policy intentions and policy outcomes cannot be bridged without attending to the constraints of profoundly racialized social, economic, and political systems.

▪ ▪ ▪

Jamila Michener is assistant professor in the Department of Government at Cornell University. She studies the politics of poverty, racial inequality, and public policy in the United States. She is author of *Fragmented Democracy: Medicaid, Federalism, and Unequal Politics* (2018). Prior to working at Cornell, she was a Robert Wood Johnson Health Policy Scholar at the University of Michigan. She received her PhD from the University of Chicago.
jm2362@cornell.edu

References

Andrulis, Dennis, Nadia J. Siddiqui, Maria R. Cooper, and Lauren R. Jahnke. 2013. "Report No. 3: Enhancing and Diversifying the Nation's Health Care Workforce." Texas Health Institute, September. www.texashealthinstitute.org/uploads/1/3/5/3/13535548/aca_workforce_report_draft_09_13_2013_final_exec_sum.pdf.

Andrulis, Dennis, Nadia J. Siddiqui, Jonathan Purtle, and Lisa Duchon. 2010. "Patient Protection and Affordable Care Act of 2010: Advancing Health Equity for Racially and Ethnically Diverse Populations." Joint Center for Political and Economic Studies, July. www.healthmanagement.com//wp-content/uploads/PPACAandDiverse Populations.pdf.

Artiga, Samantha, Anthony Damico, and Rachel Garfield. 2015. "The Impact of the Coverage Gap for Adults in States Not Expanding Medicaid by Race and Ethnicity." Kaiser Family Foundation, October 26. www.kff.org/disparities-policy /issue-brief/the-impact-of-the-coverage gap in states-not-expanding-medicaid-by -race-and-ethnicity/.

Artiga, Samantha, Kendal Orgera, and Anthony Damico. 2019. "Changes in Health Coverage by Race and Ethnicity Since Implementation of the ACA, 2013–2017." Kaiser Family Foundation, February 13. www.kff.org/disparities-policy/issue -brief/changes-in-health-coverage-by-race-and-ethnicity-since-implementation-of -the-aca-2013-2017/.

Banks, Antoine J. 2014. "The Public's Anger: White Racial Attitudes and Opinions toward Health Care Reform." *Political Behavior* 36, no. 3: 493–514.

Barrilleaux, Charles, and Carlisle Rainey. 2014. "The Politics of Need: Examining Governors' Decisions to Oppose the 'Obamacare' Medicaid Expansion." *State Politics and Policy Quarterly* 14, no. 4: 437–60.

Batalova, Jeanne, and Jie Zong. 2016. "Language Diversity and English Proficiency in the United States." Migration Policy Institute, November 11. www.migrationpolicy .org/article/language-diversity-and-english-proficiency-united-states#Age,_Race,_ and_Ethnicity.

Béland, Daniel, Philip Rocco, and Alex Waddan. 2015. "Polarized Stakeholders and Institutional Vulnerabilities: The Enduring Politics of the Patient Protection and Affordable Care Act." *Clinical Therapeutics* 37, no. 4: 720–26.

Berchick, Edward R., Jessica C. Barnett, and Rachel D. Upton. 2019. "Health Insurance Coverage in the United States: 2018." US Census Bureau, November. www .census.gov/content/dam/Census/library/publications/2019/demo/p60–267.pdf.

Bertrand, Marianne, and Sendhil Mullainathan. 2004. "Are Emily and Greg More Employable than Lakisha and Jamal? A Field Experiment on Labor Market Discrimination." *American Economic Review* 94, no. 4: 991–1013.

Bonilla-Silva, Eduardo. 1997. "Rethinking Racism: Toward a Structural Interpretation." *American Sociological Review* 62, no. 3: 465–80.

Brantley, Erin, Drishti Pillai, and Leighton Ku. 2019. "The Effects of SNAP Work Requirements and Implications for Medicaid." Paper presented at the conference "Factors Affecting Enrollment in Public Programs," AcademyHealth annual research meeting, Washington, DC, June 2. academyhealth.confex.com/academy health/2019arm/meetingapp.cgi/Paper/33443.

Bristow, Lonnie R., Adrienne Stith Butler, and Brian D. Smedley, eds. 2004. *In the Nation's Compelling Interest: Ensuring Diversity in the Healthcare Workforce.* Washington, DC: National Academies Press.

Brown, Michael K. 2003. "Ghettos, Fiscal Federalism, and Welfare Reform." In *Race and the Politics of Welfare Reform*, edited by Sanford F. Schram, Joe Soss, and Richard C. Fording, 47–71. Ann Arbor: University of Michigan Press.

Brown-Iannuzzi, Jazmin L., Erin Cooley, Stephanie E. McKee, and Charly Hyden. 2019. "Wealthy Whites and Poor Blacks: Implicit Associations between Racial Groups and Wealth Predict Explicit Opposition toward Helping the Poor." *Journal of Experimental Social Psychology* 82: 26–34.

Buchmueller, Thomas C., Zachary M. Levinson, Helen G. Levy, and Barbara L. Wolfe. 2016. "Effect of the Affordable Care Act on Racial and Ethnic Disparities in Health Insurance Coverage." *American Journal of Public Health* 106, no. 8: 1416–21.

Burwell, Sylvia Mathews. 2014. "Improving the Identification of Health Care Disparities in Medicaid and CHIP." Department of Health and Human Services, November. www.medicaid.gov/medicaid/quality-of-care/downloads/4302b-rtc-2014 .pdf.

Callaghan, Timothy, and Lawrence R. Jacobs. 2016. "Interest Group Conflict over Medicaid Expansion: The Surprising Impact of Public Advocates." *American Journal of Public Health* 106, no. 2: 308–13.

Chaudry, Ajay, Adlan Jackson, and Sherry A. Glied. 2019. "Did the Affordable Care Act Reduce Racial and Ethnic Disparities in Health Insurance Coverage?" Common Wealth Foundation, Issue Brief, August 21. www.commonwealthfund.org/publicat ions/issue-briefs/2019/aug/did-ACA-reduce-racial-ethnic-disparities-coverage.

Chen, Jie, Arturo Vargas-Bustamante, Karoline Mortensen, and Alexander N. Ortega. 2016. "Racial and Ethnic Disparities in Health Care Access and Utilization under the Affordable Care Act." *Medical Care* 54, no. 2: 140.

Delaney, Arthur, and Ariel Edwards-Levy. 2018. "Americans Are Mistaken about Who Gets Welfare." *HuffPost*, February 5. www.huffpost.com/entry/americans -welfare-perceptions-survey_n_5a7880cde4b0d3df1d13f60b.

DHHS (Department of Health and Human Services). n.d. "Putting America's Health First: FY 2020 President's Budget for HHS." www.hhs.gov/sites/default/files/fy -2020-budget-in-brief.pdf (accessed February 11, 2020).

Dovidio, John F., and Susan T. Fiske. 2012. "Under the Radar: How Unexamined Biases in Decision-Making Processes in Clinical Interactions Can Contribute to Health Care Disparities." *American Journal of Public Health* 102, no. 5: 945–52.

Fiscella, Kevin. 2016. "Why Do So Many White Americans Oppose the Affordable Care Act?" *American Journal of Medicine* 129, no. 5: e27.

Gilens, Martin. 1999. *Why Americans Hate Welfare: Race, Media, and the Politics of Antipoverty Policy*. Chicago: University of Chicago Press.

Gillion, Daniel Q. 2016. *Governing with Words: The Political Dialogue on Race, Public Policy, and Inequality in America*. New York: Cambridge University Press.

Gotham, Kevin Fox. 2000. "Racialization and the State: The Housing Act of 1934 and the Creation of the Federal Housing Administration." *Sociological Perspectives* 43, no. 2: 291–317.

Grogan, Colleen M., and Sunggeun Ethan Park. 2017. "The Racial Divide in State Medicaid Expansions." *Journal of Health Politics, Policy and Law* 42, no. 3: 539– 72.

Gutierrez, Carmen M. 2018. "The Institutional Determinants of Health Insurance: Moving Away from Labor Market, Marriage, and Family Attachments under the ACA." *American Sociological Review* 83, no. 6: 1144–70.

Hall, Garrett, and Sahai Burrowes. 2019. "Assessing the Potential Impact of Medicaid Work Requirements on African-Americans via a Welfare Reform Analysis: A Systematic Review." Cold Spring Harbor Laboratory, BioRxiv, February 13. doi.org/10.1101/549493.

Jacobs, Lawrence R., and Timothy Callaghan. 2013. "Why States Expand Medicaid: Party, Resources, and History." *Journal of Health Politics, Policy and Law* 38, no. 5: 1023–50.

KFF (Kaiser Family Foundation). n.d. "Distribution of the Nonelderly with Medicaid by Race/Ethnicity." State Health Facts. www.kff.org/medicaid/state-indicator/dis tribution-by-raceethnicity-4/?currentTimeframe=0&sortModel=%7B%22colId% 22:%22Location%22,%22sort%22:%22asc%22%7D (accessed February 11, 2020).

King, Desmond. 2017. "Forceful Federalism against American Racial Inequality." *Government and Opposition* 52, no. 2: 356–82.

Knowles, Eric D., Brian S. Lowery, and Rebecca L. Schaumberg. 2010. "Racial Prejudice Predicts Opposition to Obama and His Health Care Reform Plan." *Journal of Experimental Social Psychology* 46 no. 2: 420–23.

Lanford, Daniel, and Jill Quadagno. 2015. "Implementing ObamaCare: The Politics of Medicaid Expansion under the Affordable Care Act of 2010." *Sociological Perspectives* 59, no. 3: 619–39.

Lewis, Angela K., Pearl K. Ford Dowe, and Sekou M. Franklin. 2013. "African Americans and Obama's Domestic Policy Agenda: A Closer Look at Deracialization, the Federal Stimulus Bill, and the Affordable Care Act." *Polity* 45, no. 1: 127–52.

Lieberman, Robert C., and John S. Lapinski. 2001. "American Federalism, Race, and the Administration of Welfare." *British Journal of Political Science* 31, no. 2: 303–29.

Lipton, Brandy J., Sandra L. Decker, and Benjamin D. Sommers. 2019. "The Affordable Care Act Appears to Have Narrowed Racial and Ethnic Disparities in Insurance Coverage and Access to Care among Young Adults." *Medical Care Research and Review* 76, no. 1: 32–55.

Lowndes, Joseph E., Julie Novkov, and Dorian T. Warren, eds. 2008. *Race and American Political Development.* New York: Routledge.

Maxwell, Angie, and Todd Shields. 2014. "The Fate of Obamacare: Racial Resentment, Ethnocentrism, and Attitudes about Healthcare Reform." *Race and Social Problems* 6, no. 4: 293–304.

McCabe, Katherine T. 2019. "The Persistence of Racialized Health Care Attitudes: Racial Attitudes among White Adults and Identity Importance among Black Adults." *Journal of Race, Ethnicity, and Politics* 4, no. 2: 378–98.

McMorrow, Stacey, Sharon K. Long, Genevieve M. Kenney, and Nathaniel Anderson. 2015. "Uninsurance Disparities Have Narrowed for Black and Hispanic Adults under the Affordable Care Act." *Health Affairs* 34, no. 10: 1774–78.

Michener, Jamila. 2018. *Fragmented Democracy: Medicaid, Federalism, and Unequal Politics.* New York: Cambridge University Press.

Michener, Jamila. 2019. "Policy Feedback in a Racialized Polity." *Policy Studies Journal* 47, no. 2: 423–50.

Miller, Lisa L. 2008. *The Perils of Federalism: Race, Poverty, and the Politics of Crime Control.* New York: Oxford University Press.

Mitchell, Felicia M. 2015. "Racial and Ethnic Health Disparities in an Era of Health Care Reform." *Health and Social Work* 40, no. 3: e66–e74.

Mitchell, Joshua L., and Pearl K. Ford Dowe. 2019. "Dissecting Perceptions: Exploring the Determinants of Health-Care Reform Preferences." *Social Science Quarterly* 100, no. 1: 245–58.

Morone, James A. 2018. "Health Policy and White Nationalism: Historical Lessons, Disruptive Populism, and Two Parties at a Crossroads." *Journal of Health Politics, Policy and Law* 43, no. 4: 683–706.

National Archives. n.d. "Document Search": ACA 4302. *Federal Register.* www .federalregister.gov/documents/search?conditions%5Bterm%5D=ACA+4302.

National Archives. 2019. "Nondiscrimination in Health and Health Education Programs or Activities." *Federal Register*, June 19. www.federalregister.gov/documents/2019 /06/14/2019-11512/nondiscrimination-in-health-and-health-education-programs-or -activities.

Newkirk, Vann. 2016. "America's Health Segregation Problem: Has the Country Done Enough to Overcome Its Jim Crow Health Care History?" *Atlantic*, May 18. www .theatlantic.com/politics/archive/2016/05/americas-health-segregation-problem /483219/.

Ng, Judy H., Faye Ye, Lauren M. Ward, Samuel C. Haffer, and Sarah Hudson Scholle. 2017. "Data on Race, Ethnicity, and Language Largely Incomplete for Managed Care Plan Members." *Health Affairs* 36, no. 3: 548–52.

Ossei-Owusu, Shaun. 2016. "Racial Horizons and Empirical Landscapes in the Post-ACA World." *Wisconsin Law Review* 3: 493–514.

Pager, Devah. 2008. *Marked: Race, Crime, and Finding Work in an Era of Mass Incarceration*. Chicago: University of Chicago Press.

Pager, Devah, Bart Bonikowski, and Bruce Western. 2009. "Discrimination in a Low-Wage Labor Market: A Field Experiment." *American Sociological Review* 74, no. 5: 777–99.

Park, John J., Sarah Humble, Benjamin D. Sommers, Graham A. Colditz, Arnold M. Epstein, and Howard K. Koh. 2018. "Health Insurance for Asian Americans, Native Hawaiians, and Pacific Islanders under the Affordable Care Act." *JAMA Internal Medicine* 178, no. 8: 1128–29.

Riker, William H. 1964. *Federalism: Origin, Operation, Significance*. Boston: Little, Brown, and Company.

Sommers, Benjamin D., Anna L. Goldman, Robert J. Blendon, E. John Orav, and Arnold M. Epstein. 2019. "Medicaid Work Requirements—Results from the First Year in Arkansas." *New England Journal of Medicine* 381: 1073–82.

Soss, Joe, Richard C. Fording, and Sanford F. Schram. 2011. *Disciplining the Poor: Neoliberal Paternalism and the Persistent Power of Race*. Chicago: University of Chicago Press.

Tani, Karen M. 2016. *States of Dependency: Welfare, Rights, and American Governance, 1935–1972*. New York: Cambridge University Press.

Tesler, Michael. 2012. "The Spillover of Racialization into Health Care: How President Obama Polarized Public Opinion by Racial Attitudes and Race." *American Journal of Political Science* 56, no. 3: 690–704.

Ulmer, Cheryl, Bernadette McFadden, and David R., Nerenz, eds. 2009. *Race, Ethnicity, and Language Data: Standardization for Health Care Quality Improvement*. Washington, DC: National Academies Press.

Wagner, Jennifer, and Jessica Schubel. 2019. "States' Experiences Confirming Harmful Effects of Medicaid Work Requirements." Center on Budget and Policy Priorities, October 22. www.cbpp.org/sites/default/files/atoms/files/12-18-18health.pdf.

Wilson, Valerie. 2019. "Black Unemployment Is at Least Twice as High as White Unemployment at the National Level and in Fourteen States and the District of Columbia." Economic Policy Institute, April 4. www.epi.org/publication/valerie-figures-state-unemployment-by-race/.

Yue, Dahai, Petra W. Rasmussen, and Ninez A. Ponce. 2018. "Racial/Ethnic Differential Effects of Medicaid Expansion on Health Care Access." *Health Services Research* 53, no. 5: 3640–56.

Race, Policy Feedbacks, and Political Resilience

The Affordable Care Act and Mass Policy Feedbacks

Andrea Louise Campbell
Massachusetts Institute of Technology

Abstract The Affordable Care Act (ACA) has allowed researchers to examine mass policy feedback effects—how public policies affect individuals' attitudes and political behaviors—in real time while using causal models. These efforts help address criticisms of the extant feedbacks literature and have revealed new policy feedback effects and new information on the conditions under which policy feedbacks occur. The ACA case also raises empirical and theoretical questions about the types of data needed to assess feedback effects, the magnitude of policy effects required for detection, the time frame in which feedbacks occur, and the suitability of various empirical approaches for assessing policy feedback effects. Thus, the ACA not only adds an important empirical case to the study of policy feedbacks but also helps refine policy feedback theory.

Keywords Affordable Care Act, policy feedbacks, political behavior, public opinion

For scholars of policy feedbacks, the implementation of the Affordable Care Act (ACA) held great theoretical and empirical promise. Those who study how public policies might reshape politics had an opportunity to evaluate the effects of a major new policy in real time and to employ causal methods, addressing past concerns with this body of research. The possibility that the ACA case might reveal new types of feedbacks or new mechanisms was exciting as well.

Thus far, scholars have uncovered some positive attitudinal effects: those with personal experience getting new or improved health insurance coverage are more favorable toward the law; and some positive behavioral effects: those personally affected are more likely to vote. But the effects are modest and sometimes temporary or contradictory (in some analyses

Journal of Health Politics, Policy and Law, Vol. 45, No. 4, August 2020
DOI 10.1215/03616878-8255493   © 2020 by Duke University Press

recipient political participation declines). We may need to reconsider what types of social policy benefits *can* produce feedback effects, yielding more nuanced theory.

Concerns with Policy Feedbacks Theory and the ACA's Possible Contributions

A burgeoning literature examines public policies not just as outcomes of political processes but also as inputs. Existing policies may reshape the political environment and subsequent policy making by altering the resources and interests and mobilizing capacities of political actors at both the elite and mass levels (Béland 2010; Campbell 2012). Empirical cases of mass public reactions to social welfare policy and beyond (e.g., Simonovits et al., forthcoming) have accrued, typically showing that policies have resource and "interpretive" effects (Pierson 1993) that can be positive or negative, boosting or undermining recipients' rates of political participation or altering their preferences on public policies.

Despite theoretical and empirical advances, the policy feedbacks literature has faced both limitations and criticism. One critique warns that researchers have selected on the dependent variable, looking for cases of apparent feedbacks and then reading backward into the historical record. In many cases, we know where we have ended up and we look to program parameters and experiences to explain these patterns. The ACA promised a prospective opportunity to see what happens when Americans receive new social policy benefits—a more rigorous test in which hypothesis development preceded outcome measurement, not vice versa.

A related critique is that much policy feedbacks work has utilized observational data. Scholars have tried to strengthen causal inference, using longitudinal research designs, instrumental variables models, matching techniques, and so on, but concerns about selection and other threats to inference remain. The attitudinal and behavioral effects attributed to public policies could arise instead from preexisting characteristics of the target populations. With the quasi-experimental rollout of many of its provisions, the ACA provided an opportunity for stronger causal inference.

ACA Mass Policy Feedback Effects Thus Far

Regarding political behavior feedbacks, scholars have examined three aspects of the ACA: the Medicaid expansion, the expansion of private insurance through the Health Insurance Marketplace, and the dependent care provision allowing those under 26 to remain on their parents' insurance. Most of this work has examined policy effects on voter turnout and registration, and the findings are modest and mixed. Studies using aggregate data found that the extension of insurance coverage has increased political participation, but those using individual-level data found no effect on participation.

Haselswerdt (2017) found that aggregate turnout in House races declined less from the 2012 presidential election to the 2014 midterm in states that had expanded Medicaid, compared to those that had not. Clinton and Sances (2018) compared counties in expansion and nonexpansion states sharing a border and found that voter registration and turnout among low-income citizens under 65, the target population, increased in expansion-state counties, particularly those with a high share of eligible citizens (although the turnout effect fades over time). Courtemanche, Marton, and Yelowitz (2019) examined the effect of both Medicaid expansion and private insurance expansion via the Marketplace and the individual mandate (in place until the penalty was zeroed out by the December 2017 Tax Cuts and Jobs Act). Using individual-level participation data and estimated insurance coverage, they found that the ACA's effects were small and statistically insignificant. Chattopadhyay (2017) compared political participation among those just above and below the dependent care provision age threshold and found little effect.

Scholars have speculated on the mechanisms linking the ACA and political behavior, although existing data do not permit their rigorous evaluation. One possibility is that, in providing health insurance, the ACA may improve physical health, which is associated with greater political participation (Burden et al. 2017; Gollust and Rahn 2015; Pacheco and Fletcher 2015). Or it may boost mental health diagnosis and treatment, as did the Oregon Health Plan lottery, or reduce stress and anxiety by improving low-income families' financial stability (Baicker et al. 2013), allowing them to pursue the "luxury good" of political participation (Rosenstone and Hansen 1993).

A second mechanism could be political engagement, including political interest, knowledge, and efficacy (Verba, Schlozman, and Brady 1995) or positive "interpretive effects" (Pierson 1993). Gaining insurance through the ACA might increase recipients' sense of stake in public affairs (Clinton and Sances 2018) or make recipients feel more incorporated into the polity as deserving citizens (Pierson 1993) or more grateful to government in a way that enhances civic engagement (Mettler 2005).

A third possible mechanism is mobilization. Under the 1993 National Voter Registration Act, social assistance agencies, including the health exchanges and Medicaid offices, are required to offer voter registration, which may explain increased turnout in the Medicaid expansion states (Clinton and Sances 2018). After the 2016 election ushered in unified Republican control of government and threats to repeal the ACA, grassroots groups emerged to defend the law (Gose and Skocpol 2019; Meyer and Tarrow 2018). Policy threat can boost participation among social program recipients (Campbell 2003), although even here the evidence is mixed; for example, previous Medicaid cuts, such as Tennessee's 2005 rollback, resulted in greater turnout declines in the counties with the largest disenrollment (Haselswerdt and Michener 2019).

A new feedback effect that has emerged in the ACA case is backlash. The ACA was debated, passed, and implemented during a time of great partisanship; there is a 60– to 70–point gulf between Republicans and Democrats in favorability toward the legislation. So strong are partisan feelings that take-up varies by party identification: not only do many Republicans oppose the law even if they might benefit from it (Kliff 2016), but also Republicans in need of insurance are less likely to sign up if they encounter the government interface (healthcare.gov) than a private one (healthsherpa .com) (Lerman, Sadin, and Trachtman 2017). Some of the increased political participation after ACA implementation apparently comes from those who opposed the reform (Haselswerdt 2017; McCabe 2016). In fact, Fording and Patton (forthcoming) show that public backlash in conservative Medicaid expansion states induced lawmakers to impose new forms of conditionality on Medicaid receipt, such as work requirements, and that such policies are spreading even to states that did not expand Medicaid to begin with.

Policy feedback scholars have also examined whether implementation of the ACA would change attitudes toward the law. Perhaps favorability would rise once people gained insurance through its provisions (Jacobs and Mettler 2011) and once others realized that the worst predictions of the law's detractors did not materialize. At the same time, there were reasons to believe implementation would not change attitudes. Earlier reforms of welfare and Medicare had failed to alter attitudes, among either beneficiaries or the broader public (Morgan and Campbell 2011; Soss and Schram 2007). Partisanship often overwhelms personal experience to begin with as a factor in public preferences, and the highly partisan environment surrounding the ACA may have heightened that effect (Patashnik and Zelizer 2013). In addition, the law's complex and often hidden design elements might undermine the possibilities for attitudinal change (Chattopadhyay 2018, 2019).

Prior to implementation, symbolic factors such as partisanship, racial attitudes, and government trust dominated ACA attitudes. During the 2009–10 debate, party identification was more important in determining support or opposition to the reform than were demographic factors suggesting a material stake, including age, income, or race (Kriner and Reeves 2014). Racial attitudes were also highly correlated with ACA support (Henderson and Hillygus 2011; Tesler 2012). Panel data from the 2010–14 preimplementation period similarly showed that Republicans and those with low trust in government were more likely to say that the ACA was increasing their tax burden (Jacobs and Mettler 2016, 2018).

After implementation began, modest evidence of increased support among those benefiting from the law's provisions—an attitudinal policy feedback—emerged. Fewer survey respondents said the law had no effect on health care access (Jacobs and Mettler 2016). The gap between Republicans and Democrats in ACA favorability was smaller among those who gained insurance through the Marketplace than among those with employer-based insurance (McCabe 2016). Between 2010 and 2017, Medicaid expansion made lower-income Americans more favorable toward the ACA, with effects stronger among nonwhites and Democrats (Hopkins and Parish, forthcoming). Those with personal or family experience gaining insurance, using subsidies, or getting prescription drug help as senior citizens were more likely to say the ACA has had a favorable impact on health access (Jacobs and Mettler 2018). Those buying insurance in the Marketplace were more positive toward the ACA than those who remained uninsured, as were those in their early sixties whose insurance premiums were newly capped by the law (Hobbs and Hopkins 2019). At the same time, those purchasing insurance on the exchanges who experienced local premium spikes became less favorable toward the ACA (Hobbs and Hopkins 2019).

The political environment mattered—pro-ACA announcements by governors in one state increased public support for the law in nearby states (Pacheco and Maltby 2017)—as did political threat: pooled 2009–17 data showed that after the 2016 election made Republican repeal threats credible, ACA approval was higher (and support for repeal lower) in Medicaid expansion states compared to nonexpansion states, especially among lower-education nonsenior adults (Sances and Clinton 2019).

Thus, evidence both from panel surveys (Jacobs and Mettler 2016) and causal analyses (Hobbs and Hopkins 2019; Sances and Clinton 2019) shows that personal experience altered attitudes toward the ACA. In some instances, the benefits conferred are tangible, visible, and large enough (Citrin and Green 1991) to enhance political participation and to induce protective stances, especially in the face of policy threat. And the ACA has highlighted a previously unrecognized phenomenon, political backlash, useful for explaining greater participation by a law's opponents. That said, in many instances these feedback effects are small in magnitude, contradictory in direction, and in some cases, temporary.

Why Haven't More Feedbacks Emerged?

Scholars have begun to speculate about the modest size of policy feedbacks arising from the ACA. The ACA's hidden design elements—using private insurance to spread coverage in the Marketplace, in the dependent coverage provision, in Medicaid managed care—makes it difficult for recipients to connect their health insurance experience to government activity, undercutting attitudinal or behavioral change (Chattopadhyay 2018, 2019; see also Béland, Rocco, and Waddan 2019). The facts that important policy decisions were devolved to the state level and that some state implementation choices increased public support for the ACA while others decreased it suggest that federalism can undermine policy feedbacks (Pacheco and Maltby 2019). Another possibility is that, while the vociferous public debate over the ACA may have enhanced feedback effects by informing people about the law, it may also have heightened the influence of partisanship and motivated reasoning over personal experience as a factor in attitudes and behaviors around the law (Patashnik and Zelizer 2013). Because the ACA's target populations—low-income or young in many cases—are marginal voters to begin with, the benefits may have been insufficient to push them permanently over the participatory hump, explaining why some of the participation increases have been only temporary (Clinton and Sances 2018). Oberlander and Weaver (2015) argued the ACA has suffered "self-undermining policy feedbacks" for reasons like those above, which concern beneficiaries themselves, as well as additional factors, such as concentrated losses and festering grievances among significant groups like taxpayers and employers, persistent political incentives for key elites to criticize the law's provisions and characterize its beneficiaries as undeserving, and the law's vulnerability to legal challenge.

These observations strike me as correct, but I believe ACA feedback effects have been modest for additional reasons. Some of these factors are specific to the ACA or to health policy. Yet others have larger theoretical and empirical implications for policy feedbacks scholarship.

First, we may be looking at the wrong political acts. Most analyses of behavioral feedbacks have focused on voter registration and turnout, the acts that are the most common and have the best data availability. But voting is driven not just by resources but especially by civic duty (Verba, Schlozman, and Brady 1995), so it may not be the most sensitive instrument for assessing a resource effect arising from a new social policy benefit. The vote is also a blunt instrument with little information-carrying capacity (Verba, Schlozman, and Brady 1995). Political acts that are more policy specific, such as contacting elected officials or protest, may be better measures of policy feedback. Anecdotal evidence suggests that Republicans' ACA repeal attempts spurred protest activity (e.g., Gose and Skocpol 2019), but we lack the data to systematically assess that possibility, hence scholars' emphasis so far on voting.

Second, it may be that the ACA is simply less capable of producing policy feedback effects than are other policies. To Chattopadhyay's points about the ACA's fractured design undermining possible feedback effects, I add the visibility of fellow recipients. That the ACA provides different policy fixes for different types of people getting health insurance from different sources undermines the proximity and visibility that seem to fuel some feedback effects. Consider senior citizens receiving Social Security and Medicare. They can readily recognize one another. They are also numerous, located everywhere, and in some places even live together. But ACA beneficiaries cannot identify each other. Some get health insurance because they are newly eligible for Medicaid, some because they were previously eligible but newly signed up, some because they are newly purchasing private plans on exchanges, with or without government subsidies, and some because they can stay on their parents' private health insurance until age 26. Such individuals are scattered everywhere, concentrated nowhere. There are few mechanisms—either through the programs themselves or through mobilizing organizations, which barely exist—for such individuals to recognize one another and work together. Such organizations are crucial for both asking people to participate and explaining to them the stakes of public debates. Even if mobilizing organizations were to emerge, they would have difficulty identifying potential members. Health politics may be unique because health has a private cast that may undermine public efforts at mobilization and because health concerns often do not align with other forms of identity (Carpenter 2012). On top of those complicating factors, the ACA's fractured policy design heightens informational and mobilizational barriers.

A third and related point is that the ACA may be less likely to create feedback effects because its benefits are too modest and its policy mechanisms too indirect. Consider Social Security: The program's retirement benefits are large enough to solve, mostly, the problem of senior poverty (although pockets of poverty remain, especially among women, ethnic and racial minorities, and older seniors). They also address the underlying problem of retirement security directly, with cash delivered to the household budget. Or consider food stamps: They vary in size with income, and even the maximum benefit was never intended to cover 100% of recipients' food purchases. The mechanism, however, is direct: an EBT card that is used to purchase food, alleviating hunger.

In contrast, consider health insurance: What people really want is health security—access to affordable health insurance and medical care—but the ACA falls short of its promise for many, solving so little of the underlying problem.[1] One shortcoming is the magnitude of its benefits: the subsidies on the exchanges are too small to make insurance affordable for many, and the law has failed to stem rising deductibles and underinsurance in the employer market. Inadequate health insurance means continued health insecurity for many Americans. The other problem is the indirectness of the mechanism, a phenomenon inherent to health insurance, not just the ACA. Compared to a direct mechanism like injecting cash or cash equivalents into the household budget, health insurance provides financial security more indirectly. Ideally health insurance is complete enough not to cripple households' budgets with unaffordable out-of-pocket costs; ideally health insurance provides sufficient access to health care to support work or whatever activity makes for the household budget. But both of these linkages between health insurance and financial security are probabilistic. The more a program falls short of its goals, whether through the inadequacy of the benefit or the indirectness of its mechanism, the less its feedback-generating capacity.

Fourth, it is worth underlining the effects of heightened partisanship and polarization on the ACA's ability to generate feedback effects (Oberlander and Weaver 2015; Patashnik and Zelizer 2013). Ordinary people, for whom politics and policy are a sideshow in life, need help interpreting political events and policy changes. High levels of partisanship and polarization mean the public has been continually bombarded with conflicting messages on the ACA from elites, including a highly critical stream from the political Right. The benefits of the ACA are thus disputed in the public

---

1. Thanks to Jon Oberlander for his comments on this paragraph.

realm, likely undermining the development of support among beneficiaries, whose personal experience is tarnished, and among nonbeneficiaries, who, lacking personal experience, were suspicious to begin with. It is easier for a reform to become the new normal when elite messages are more consistently supportive.

Fifth, and most important for policy feedbacks theory, is the role of time. Feedback effects may be modest thus far because of the relatively short time the ACA has been in existence. If the linkage between the ACA and increased political activity is the resource of improved health then it could take years for improved health to materialize, as the Oregon Health Plan experience suggests (Baicker et al. 2013).

More profoundly, thinking about time raises some serious questions about the use of causal models—or at least the types of causal models we have been using—to detect feedback effects. The ACA has facilitated the causal analysis of policy feedback effects, which I applaud. But many causal models presume immediate effects: recipients get a new benefit, and now they instantly have new interests, or they instantly receive and internalize "interpretive" messages about their worth as citizens that should influence their attitudes and behaviors in the short term. That is, many extant causal models presume a type of flip-the-switch effect. But is that what happens? Do we really think that people adopt a new set of interests, or recognize a new set of citizenship messages, that quickly? Some factors can change in the short term, such as the resource factors feeding into political participation. But other factors underlying political participation and especially political attitudes are less conducive to immediate change. Something else to ponder: we know that aggregate opinion change typically comes about through cohort replacement, not individual-level change, which suggests the flip-the-switch effect may be rare indeed.[2]

Moreover, the short time frame of many causal models measures only the "feed," not the "back," and hence does not encapsulate a complete expression of policy feedbacks theory. If we think that feedbacks happen in a cyclical, iterative fashion, with policies changing attitudes and behaviors, which in turn reverberate through the political system to produce new policies, then causal models may capture only one-half of one iteration of the cycle, too short term to capture the full phenomenon. In addition, some mechanisms connecting a policy with political behaviors and attitudes may take longer to materialize than others. Consider my analysis of the role of Social Security in boosting senior citizens' political participation, which

2. Many thanks to Julianna Pacheco for this observation.

showed that these effects grew iteratively over decades (Campbell 2003). It took time for the resource effect to grow, as more seniors were eligible for retirement benefits and as they grew more generous. It took time for mobilizing entities to focus on seniors as a political constituency worthy of outreach efforts. It took even more time for seniors' outsized sense of political efficacy to develop, as they observed their bursts of participation aimed at protecting the program recognized and rewarded by politicians. Clearly causal models deserve a place in policy feedbacks work—we must know that an effect we observe is truly due to the policy itself and not competing factors—but we must also recognize the limits of causal models and utilize them in conjunction with other methods of assessing the relationships between public policies and public behaviors and attitudes over time.

Future Research in Mass Policy Feedbacks

The ACA has added an important case of policy feedback, providing a new example of threat as a motivator and revealing a new phenomenon—backlash—to look for in other policy areas. We see yet again the toll that obscured, complicated policy designs (especially privatized designs) take on individuals' ability to recognize the government role in their public policy experiences and to defend it. And we have the welcome extension of causal models to this empirical area, where they have been sorely needed.

But the ACA case also shows that scholars of policy feedback still have work to do. We need to think more deeply about what causal models imply about the timing and nature of policy feedbacks. We need more data, both survey data and qualitative data, that follow individuals' program experiences and evolving thinking and behavior and that follows mobilizing organizations and their strategies. As always, we need more analyses that show both that policies influence attitudes and behaviors and that, in turn, those altered attitudes and behaviors reshape the political environment and influence subsequent rounds of policymaking. In this regard I commend the work of Fording and Patton (forthcoming), which shows that Medicaid expansion by Republican governors angered Republican voters in their states (the feed), which induced those governors to impose work requirements to retroactively limit Medicaid expansion (the back). And "the back" has continued: states newly adopting Medicaid expansion have decided to impose work requirements from the outset, and even states that never adopted Medicaid expansion have decided to impose work requirements on their existing programs. This scholarship confirms the value of the policy feedback approach, which I hope the ACA—the most important social policy change in a generation—will continue to foster.

▪ ▪ ▪

Andrea Louise Campbell is Sloan Professor of Political Science at MIT. Her interests include American politics, political behavior, public opinion, political inequality, and policy feedbacks. She is the author of *How Policies Make Citizens: Senior Citizen Activism and the American Welfare State* (2003), *The Delegated Welfare State: Medicare, Markets, and the Governance of Social Policy*, with Kimberly J. Morgan (2011), and *Trapped in America's Safety Net: One Family's Struggle* (2014). She is a member of the American Academy of Arts and Sciences.
acampbel@mit.edu

Acknowledgments

I thank Jon Oberlander, Julianna Pacheco, and Jacqueline Chattopadhyay for their very helpful comments on an earlier version of the manuscript.

References

Baicker, Katherine, Sarah L. Taubman, Heidi L. Allen, Mira Bernstein, Jonathan H. Gruber, Joseph P. Newhouse, Eric C. Schneider, Bill J. Wright, Alan M. Zaslavsky, and Amy N. Finkelstein. 2013. "The Oregon Experiment—Effects of Medicaid on Clinical Outcomes." *New England Journal of Medicine* 368: 1713–22.

Béland, Daniel. 2010. "Reconsidering Policy Feedback: How Policies Affect Politics." *Administration and Society* 42, no. 5: 568–90.

Béland, Daniel, Philip Rocco, and Alex Waddan. 2019. "Policy Feedback and the Politics of the Affordable Care Act." *Policy Studies Journal* 47, no. 2: 395–422.

Burden, Barry C., Jason M. Fletcher, Pamela Herd, Donald P. Moynihan, and Bradley M. Jones. 2017. "How Different Forms of Health Matter to Political Participation." *Journal of Politics* 79, no. 1: 166–78.

Campbell, Andrea Louise. 2003. *How Policies Make Citizens: Senior Citizen Activism and the American Welfare State.* Princeton, NJ: Princeton University Press.

Campbell, Andrea Louise. 2012. "Policy Makes Mass Politics." *Annual Review of Political Science* 15: 333–51.

Carpenter, Daniel. 2012. "Is Health Politics Different?" *Annual Review of Political Science* 15: 287–311.

Chattopadhyay, Jacqueline. 2017. "Is the ACA's Dependent Coverage Provision Generating Positive Feedback Effects among Young Adults?" *Poverty and Public Policy* 9, no. 1: 42–70.

Chattopadhyay, Jacqueline. 2018. "Is the Affordable Care Act Cultivating a Cross-Class Constituency? Income, Partisanship, and a Proposal for Tracing the Contingent Nature of Positive Policy Feedback Effects." *Journal of Health Politics, Policy and Law* 43, no. 1: 19–67.

Chattopadhyay, Jacqueline. 2019. "Can Health Insurance Regulations Generate Citizen Constituencies?" *Journal of Health Politics, Policy and Law* 44, no. 3: 455–78.

Citrin, Jack, and Donald P. Green. 1991. "The Self-Interest Motive in American Public Opinion." In *Research in Micropolitics*, edited by Samuel Long, 1–28. Greenwich, CT: JIA.

Clinton, Joshua D., and Michael W. Sances. 2018. "The Politics of Policy: The Initial Mass Political Effects of Medicaid Expansion in the States." *American Political Science Review* 112, no. 1: 167–85.

Courtemanche, Charles, James Marton, and Aaron Yelowitz. 2019. "The Full Impact of the Affordable Care Act on Political Participation." Paper presented at the Russell Sage Foundation, New York, NY, May 29.

Fording, Richard C., and Dana Patton. Forthcoming. "The Affordable Care Act and the Diffusion of Policy Feedback: The Case of Medicaid Work Requirements." Paper presented at the Russell Sage Foundation, New York, NY, May 29.

Gollust, Sarah E., and Wendy M. Rahn. 2015. "The Bodies Politic: Chronic Health Conditions and Voter Turnout in the 2008 Election." *Journal of Health Politics, Policy and Law* 40, no. 6: 1115–55.

Gose, Leah, and Theda Skocpol. 2019. "Resist, Persist, and Transform: The Emergence and Impact of Grassroots Resistance Groups Opposing the Trump Presidency." Working paper, Harvard University, March 21. scholar.harvard.edu/files/thedaskocpol/files/resist_persist_and_transform_3–21–19_.ap_.pdf.

Haselswerdt, Jake. 2017. "Expanding Medicaid, Expanding the Electorate: The Affordable Care Act's Short-Term Impact on Political Participation." *Journal of Health Politics, Policy and Law* 42, no. 4: 667–95.

Haselswerdt, Jake, and Jamila Michener. 2019. "Disenrolled: Retrenchment and Voting in Health Policy." *Journal of Health Politics, Policy and Law* 44, no. 3: 423–54.

Henderson, Michael, and D. Sunshine Hillygus. 2011. "The Dynamics of Health Care Opinion, 2008–2010: Partisanship, Self-Interest, and Racial Resentment." *Journal of Health Politics, Policy and Law* 36, no. 6: 945–60.

Hobbs, William R., and Daniel J. Hopkins. 2019. "Offsetting Policy Feedback Effects: Evidence from the Affordable Care Act." SSRN, July 5. ssrn.com/abstract=3366994.

Hopkins, Daniel J., and Kalind Parish. 2019. "The Medicaid Expansion and Attitudes toward the Affordable Care Act: Testing for a Policy Feedback on Mass Opinion." *Public Opinion Quarterly* 83, no. 1: 123–34.

Jacobs, Lawrence R., and Suzanne Mettler. 2011. "Why Public Opinion Changes: The Implications for Health and Health Policy." *Journal of Health Politics, Policy and Law* 36, no. 6: 917–33.

Jacobs, Lawrence R., and Suzanne Mettler. 2016. "Liking Health Reform but Turned Off by Toxic Politics." *Health Affairs* 35, no. 5: 915–22.

Jacobs, Lawrence R., and Suzanne Mettler. 2018. "When and How New Policy Creates New Politics: Examining the Feedback Effects of the Affordable Care Act on Public Opinion." *Perspectives on Politics* 16, no. 2: 345–63.

Kliff, Sarah. 2016. "Why Obamacare Enrollees Voted for Trump." *Vox*, December 13. www.vox.com/science-and-health/2016/12/13/13848794/kentucky-obamacare -trump.

Kriner, Douglas L., and Andrew Reeves. 2014. "Responsive Partisanship: Public Support for the Clinton and Obama Health Care Plans." *Journal of Health Politics, Policy and Law* 39, no. 4: 717–49.

Lerman, Amy E., Meredith L. Sadin, and Samuel Trachtman. 2017. "Policy Uptake as Political Behavior: Evidence from the Affordable Care Act." *American Political Science Review* 111, no. 4: 755–70.

McCabe, Katherine T. 2016. "Attitude Responsiveness and Partisan Bias: Direct Experience with the Affordable Care Act." *Political Behavior* 38, no. 4: 861–82.

Mettler, Suzanne. 2005. *Soldiers to Citizens: The G.I. Bill and the Making of the Greatest Generation*. New York: Oxford University Press.

Meyer, David S., and Sidney Tarrow. 2018. *The Resistance: The Dawn of the Anti-Trump Opposition Movement*. New York: Oxford University Press.

Morgan, Kimberly J., and Andrea Louise Campbell. 2011. *The Delegated Welfare State: Medicare, Markets, and the Governance of American Social Policy*. New York: Oxford University Press.

Oberlander, Jonathan, and R. Kent Weaver. 2015. "Unraveling from Within? The Affordable Care Act and Self-Undermining Policy Feedbacks." *Forum* 13, no. 1: 37–62.

Pacheco, Julianna, and Jason Fletcher. 2015. "Incorporating Health into Studies of Political Behavior: Evidence for Turnout and Partisanship." *Political Research Quarterly* 68, no. 1: 104–16.

Pacheco, Julianna, and Elizabeth Maltby. 2017. "The Role of Public Opinion—Does It Influence the Diffusion of ACA Decisions?" *Journal of Health Politics, Policy and Law* 42, no. 2: 309–40.

Pacheco, Julianna, and Elizabeth Maltby. 2019. "Trends in State-Level Opinion toward the Affordable Care Act." *Journal of Health Politics, Policy and Law* 44, no. 5: 737–64.

Patashnik, Eric M., and Julian E. Zelizer. 2013. "The Struggle to Remake Politics: Liberal Reform and the Limits of Policy Feedback in the Contemporary American State." *Perspectives on Politics* 11, no. 4: 1071–87.

Pierson, Paul. 1993. "When Effect Becomes Cause: Policy Feedback and Political Change." *World Politics* 45, no. 4: 595–628.

Rosenstone, Steven J., and John Mark Hansen. 1993. *Mobilization, Participation, and Democracy in America*. New York: Macmillan.

Sances, Michael W., and Joshua D. Clinton. 2019. "Policy Effects, Partisanship, and Elections: How Medicaid Expansion Affected Opinions of the Affordable Care Act." Working paper, November. sites.temple.edu/msances/research/.

Simonovits, Gabor, Neil Malhotra, Raymond Ye Lee, and Andrew Healy. 2019. "The Effect of Distributive Politics on Electoral Participation: Evidence from 70 Million

Agricultural Payments." *Political Behavior*, October 15. link.springer.com/article /10.1007/s11109-019-09572-7.

Soss, Joe, and Sanford F. Schram. 2007. "A Public Transformed? Welfare Reform as Policy Feedback." *American Political Science Review* 101, no. 1: 111–27.

Tesler, Michael. 2012. "The Spillover of Racialization into Health Care: How President Obama Polarized Public Opinion by Race and Racial Attitudes." *American Journal of Political Science* 56, no. 3: 690–704.

Verba, Sidney, Kay Lehman Schlozman, and Henry E. Brady. 1995. *Voice and Equality*. Cambridge, MA: Harvard University Press.

Race, Policy Feedbacks, and Political Resilience

What Health Reform Tells Us about American Politics

Lawrence R. Jacobs
University of Minnesota

Suzanne Mettler
Cornell University

Abstract The passage and initial implementation of the Affordable Care Act (ACA) were imperiled by partisan divisions, court challenges, and the quagmire of federalism. In the aftermath of Republican efforts to repeal the ACA, however, the law not only carries on but also is changing the nature of political debate as its benefits are facilitating increased support for it, creating new constituents who rely on its benefits and share intense attachments to them, and lifting the confidence of Americans in both their individual competence to participate effectively in politics and that government will respond. Critics from the Left and the Right differ on their favored remedy, but both have failed to appreciate the qualitative shifts brought on by the ACA; this myopia results from viewing reform as a fixed endpoint instead of a process of evolution over time. The result is that conservatives have been blind to the widening network of support for the ACA, while those on the left have underestimated health reform's impact in broadening recognition of medical care as a right of citizenship instead of a privilege earned in the workplace. The forces that constrained the ACA's development still rage in American politics, but they no longer dictate its survival as they did during its passage in 2010.

Keywords health reform, politics, partisanship

The implementation and operation of the Affordable Care Act (ACA), though tumultuous, fraught, and obstacle ridden at every stage, have nonetheless transformed the politics of health reform in the United States. Since the New Deal, American reformers had struggled uphill to guarantee health coverage to all Americans. They eventually succeeded in attaining government coverage for seniors, disabled, and certain categories of

Journal of Health Politics, Policy and Law, Vol. 45, No. 4, August 2020
DOI 10.1215/03616878-8255505   © 2020 by Duke University Press

low-income people. They failed, however, to establish national health insurance for the working-age population—until the enactment of the ACA.

It was remarkable enough for the law to be enacted, but all the more so for it to survive over the next decade. Political division and dysfunction bombarded the ACA at every turn: throughout its arduous journey through Congress to President Obama's desk, during the repeated court challenges that followed, and as much of its implementation took place amid the quagmire of federalism. The rigid partisan divide in Congress produced a party-line vote on passing the Affordable Care Act in 2009–10 and, after its passage, foreclosed possibilities for national lawmakers to create practical, technical adjustments. Partisanship in state governments slowed or stymied their efforts to shepherd the rollout of the law's programs for low- and middle-income Americans. The partisan divide also split ordinary Americans in their views about the law. The election of Donald Trump and a Republican Congress in 2016 initiated an unprecedented attack on this landmark legislation: bills to repeal the ACA passed in the US House of Representatives and came within one vote of clearing the US Senate, surviving only when Senator John McCain joined his Republican colleagues Susan Collins and Lisa Murkowski in opposing it.

The persistence of the ACA over its first decade of such formidable odds represents an immense achievement. It did not occur readily or automatically; in fact, it nearly failed at multiple junctures. Yet today, the law not only carries on but has gained greater support and generated political involvement among ordinary Americans. The ACA is increasingly changing the nature of political debate. The forces that constrained its development still rage in American politics, but they no longer dictate the ACA's survival as they did during its passage in 2010.

New policies often remain fragile during their early years; ideally, policy makers can nurture them, enacting helpful adjustments along the way and providing administrators with ample resources and other assistance to ensure success (Berry, Burden, and Howell 2012; Patashnik 2008). The ACA, however, emerged amid a firestorm in American politics, as intensifying partisan polarization and congressional gridlock fostered an environment that is inhospitable to reform. The resilience and growing strength of the ACA, even in the midst of this environment, present a puzzle that requires explanation.

Together and separately we have been tracking the topsy-turvy history of the ACA. In studies represented by a string of publications and papers, we conducted elite interviews, examined primary and secondary sources, collected multiple waves of panel data, and conducted multivariate regression analysis. While some of our findings, particularly regarding early implementation, confirm aspects of the familiar patterns associated with partisanship, lobbying by powerful interests, and legislative gridlock, we also found that these patterns did not dictate the ACA's first decade. As time went on, we found, the ACA itself generated policy feedback dynamics that have enabled it to survive and even, in some respects, to thrive. In these regards, it presents striking — if contingent — exceptions to the dynamics of contemporary American politics.

National Gridlock and State Implementation

In an unprecedented departure from the pattern followed previously by partisans of both parties when landmark legislation passed over their disapproval in Washington, DC, Republican opposition to the ACA's passage has yet to subside. Following the 2010 elections, party leaders took note of the influx of Tea Party Republicans that successfully flipped the House to Republican control and identified ACA repeal as a winning issue that mobilized their voters. This in turn produced widespread agreement among political commentators and the news media that health reform was doomed to paralysis or collapse (e.g. Boyer 2010; Edsall 2013). This narrative of doom made sense early on, but over time it has obscured immense shifts in the law's development.

Public opinion toward health reform initially followed a pattern that has become familiar in an age of polarization: Americans split into rigid partisan groupings who shared similar conservative or liberal mindsets generally, and they adopted positions of support or opposition to the ACA accordingly (Abramowitz 2010; Levendusky 2009). Such partisan sorting, according to social psychologists, results from "hot cognition," in which individuals are triggered by elite or media cues and respond with near automatic reflex (Taber and Lodge 2006).

The combination of the partisan standoff over the ACA among elected officials in Washington and polarized views about it among the public reinforced each other, producing gridlock over it in Congress. This prevented the passage of incremental adjustments and even technical legislation to fix glitches (Holahan and Blumberg 2017). Such technical fixes were familiar in the past, even after heated congressional disputes. For instance, the enactment of the Medicare Modernization Act of 2003 was fiercely contested, and yet, after it was signed by President George W. Bush, lawmakers worked together in a bipartisan manner to revise and improve the law.

The patterns of partisan polarization and gridlock that hindered the ACA in its early years broke down in the states, however, as implementation proceeded. For sure, there was a close association between early state adoption of the Medicaid expansion and Democratic control of state legislatures and especially governorships. Yet, sweeping conclusions about the ACA's prospects generated by journalists and others were typically based on the loud and vociferous conflict in Washington and among national politicians and crucially missed the cracks in partisan stalemate that were starting to appear at the state level. While partisanship remained (Republicans controlled all the states that blocked Medicaid expansion), a steady pattern commenced of GOP lawmakers adopting the new benefits.

One of the factors that contributed to the implementation of health reform by states was their strategic maneuvering to engage in intergovernmental bargaining. In an analysis of 50 states, Callaghan and Jacobs (2014) found that states with prior experience seeking federal waivers for social welfare programs made more progress toward Medicaid expansion than those lacking that track record, after controlling for party control in government. In particular, this points to the mechanism of "upward federalism" in which states that requested 1115 waivers from Medicaid before 2010 treated the ACA's original design of Medicaid expansion as an opening bid for negotiations to press for greater leeway. For federal agencies, the process of back-and-forth consultations and negotiations with interested states was welcomed as a means to identify areas of potential compromise in order to induce state adoption of the Medicaid expansion (as was the case with Arkansas's "private option"). However, states that either lacked the experience of requesting waivers or were unrelentingly opposed to implementing the ACA viewed the 2010 law as a "take-it-or-leave-it" order and refused to engage in negotiations.

Empirical research added additional explanations for the loosening grip of partisanship on state implementation of the ACA, as GOP governors in Arizona, Nevada, Michigan, and other states moved forward with the Medicaid expansion. The analysis pointed to several factors that would later prove to be significant drivers: states appeared predisposed toward expanding Medicaid if they had previously established programs to assist low-income people (what we more fully describe below as "policy feedback") or possessed the administrative capacity to manage health care programs (Jacobs and Callaghan 2013). By 2015, the partisan control of government continued to influence Medicaid expansion and, in particular, variations in new enrollment across all 50 states. But empirical evidence also continued to reveal the impact of state health policy and administrative capacity on the enrollment of individuals in Medicaid after taking into account the influence of partisanship (Callaghan and Jacobs 2017). An important pattern became evident: political parties still mattered, but they did not impose rigid control outside of Washington.

Cracks in America's Oligarchy

Rising economic inequality, along with the political organization of corporations and the affluent, has produced a reinforcing cycle of increasingly concentrated power and resources in contemporary American politics that some describe as "oligarchic" (Gilens and Page 2014; Jacobs and Page 2005; Skocpol and Hertel-Fernandez 2016). The results of lopsided organized combat are evident in tax and labor policies that advantage corporations and the wealthiest individuals.

The Obama White House launched its campaign to pass the ACA in 2009 by making concessions to the medical professions and the powerful interests associated with commercial insurers, hospital, pharmaceutical producers, and more (Jacobs and Skocpol 2015). These types of accommodations are a familiar pattern in American politics, typically present particularly when reform is attempted in a domain already populated by stakeholders. Previous efforts at health care reform failed, in part, because such groups opposed it; for example, the American Medical Association stymied the reform efforts of Presidents Franklin D. Roosevelt and Harry Truman, and the health insurance industry thwarted efforts by President Bill Clinton (Blumenthal and Morone 2010).

Nonetheless, the ACA departs, in crucial respects, from the pattern of bias toward the organized and affluent. Even though health reform contained concessions, they were granted for the purpose of its central achievement: the extension of the right to health care as a basic component of citizenship (Jacobs 2014). The ACA succeeded in bringing health insurance coverage to more than 20 million people and preventing more than 19,000 deaths due to the lack of medical care, according to one estimate (Miller et al. 2019). The law was financed predominantly through new taxes on the wealthiest Americans, including a higher Medicare tax on earnings and a new 3.8% tax on investment income (Tax Policy Center 2018). These historic gains occurred, in part, because of another departure: the dynamics of organized politics changed in several respects.

Organized interests often unify against expanding social welfare benefits for the less advantaged, fearing tax increases and new regulations that might accompany such policies. In the case of the ACA, however, such groups split, as some voiced their typical opposition but others came out as supporters. In particular, health care providers, suppliers, and segments of the insurance industry valued the law's distribution of subsidies and other benefits that increased demand for health insurance, medical care, prescription medications, and medical equipment (Hertel-Fernandez, Skocpol, and Lynch 2016; Jacobs and Ario 2012; Jacobs and Skocpol 2015). Business associations, especially the US Chamber of Commerce and the Koch network (including its conservative American Legislative Exchange Council), contested the passage and implementation of the ACA but found their resources and influence offset, in part, by medical groups and other health care stakeholders that favored the law's success.

As well-resourced business and professional organizations splintered, the public interest advocates for ACA implementation weighed in. Over 9,200 lobbyists registered in state capitols to push for their clients' preferred health policy. Callaghan and Jacobs (2016) found that states that included a greater number of lobbyists for the uninsured and vulnerable, such as those associated with unions and consumer and charitable organizations, made greater progress in implementing the ACA's Medicaid expansion by 2015 than did states that had fewer such advocates in their capitols. The positive and significant impact of public interest advocates held up even after controlling for the partisan control of state government, the well-funded pressure from businesses and professionals, and other potentially confounding factors.

The Politics That Health Reform Created

The old saw about generals is that they fight the last war with less regard for intervening changes. Political commentators following health reform have tended to fall into the same trap, assuming that the battle lines of 2009–10 would continue to define the politics surrounding the ACA going forward. Of course, they are correct with respect to the partisan split in Washington, DC, which has certainly persisted. Nonetheless, this first decade of the ACA's implementation has changed the politics of health reform, specifically with respect to Americans' attitudes and political behavior.

The Changing Public

We have been carefully tracking the reactions of everyday Americans to the ACA. As reform was moving through Congress in 2009, we set up a panel of 1,000 randomly selected American adults as well as 200 people from groups who are often underrepresented in surveys—lower income and younger people. We have interviewed this panel every other fall from 2010 through 2018, creating five waves of interviews with the same group of people. Our panel is weighted to represent US demographic characteristics and has retained many of our original interviewees.[1]

By 2014, the ACA's programs were already tarnished by administrative mishaps even though most were not yet implemented; Americans' attitudes toward health reform at this stage reflected this (Jacobs and Mettler 2018). Our analysis of the first three waves in 2010, 2012, and 2014 found that Americans were generally supportive of the ACA's specific benefits, such as subsidies to purchase private insurance or help for seniors to purchase prescription medication. As the years unfolded, there were also signs that resistance to the ACA might be receding a bit: support for outright repeal remained robust but was declining, and fewer members of our panel reported that the ACA had little or no impact on access to health care than had done so at the outset. Still, the partisan divide created a toxic environment that undermined support for health reform overall. No regular observer of American politics would be surprised to learn that Democrats favored the law and Republicans retained unfavorable views of it.

Our sustained analysis has detected an important development as the years proceeded, however: the implementation of the ACA was changing the politics of health reform, modestly at first and then more robustly by October 2018. This pattern is consistent with research on policy feedback: individuals' personal experiences with established programs and those with designs that make government's role visible can change public attitudes and political engagement, including voting behavior (Campbell 2003; Mettler 2005, 2011).

Our research found early signs of the ACA's effects on the politics of health reform. By late 2014, Americans who gained insurance coverage and saw tangible benefits of subsidies and help for seniors became, compared to their earlier atttitudes, more appreciative of the law's impact in expanding access to coverage (Jacobs and Mettler 2018).

Despite these signs of increasing appreciation of the law's specific benefits, however, our analysis of public attitudes toward it in late 2014 made evident why overall public support for the ACA generally had not yet grown (Jacobs and Mettler 2018). The ACA had created benefits, but it also introduced burdens in the form of taxes. Although the taxes fell

1. Overall, 66% (949 of 1,473) of panelists from prior waves sampled completed the wave 5 interview. Forty-four percent of the original 2010 survey (524 individuals) responded to all five waves, and 58% (691 individuals) participated in both 2010 and 2018.

predominantly on a small group of Americans in the top 1% of the income distribution, they initially contributed to antireform judgments (Tax Policy Center 2018). Partisanship and distrust of government, moreover, continued to overwhelm even Americans' positive experiences of it when it came to their overall evaluations of health reform. Compared to their assessments in 2010, individuals who identified as Republicans and resented government and taxes increased their unfavorable assessment of reform's impact on access, as did those who lost insurance coverage since the ACA's enactment. Nonetheless, the upward trend in the appreciation of the laws' features would, within the next few years, harken more fundamental shifts in public opinion and political behavior.

Four Features of the New Health Politics

When President Obama and Democrats struggled to pass health reform in 2009–10, the stakes remained vague to most Americans, as neither the scope of the benefits nor the recipients of the burdens were apparent. As the ACA reaches its 10–year anniversary, it provides concrete services and its impact on the lives of everyday Americans has become tangible—and expected. Anticipated burdens have failed to materialize for most people.

New health policy changed the politics of health reform in four respects. First, Americans have become increasingly accustomed to receiving the ACA's benefits, and that has led to growing support. The partisan frame that initially defined responses to the ACA has given way, for many Americans, to a pragmatic frame, in which more acknowledge the value of receiving needed health coverage. Panel data shows that support for the ACA increased by the fall of 2018 to its highest level since the law's enactment, and the most intense opposition had receded to its lowest point. More individuals have also been reporting that the ACA affected their lives and improved their access to health care, even after Republicans and the Trump administration attempted to undermine the law. In particular, individuals have grown more appreciative by 2018 compared with earlier years of the ACA's help for seniors to achieve prescription drug coverage, subsidies to purchase private health insurance, and guarantee of insurance for the children of insured parents until 26 years of age.

Second, the Washington GOP's threat to repeal the ACA in 2017–18—once they controlled both the White House and both chambers of Congress—jolted a broad swath of Americans to become more supportive of the law than they had been before the 2016 elections (Zhu, Mettler, and Jacobs 2019). Democrats had long been supportive of the law, but in the wake of the GOP threat, support for it increased among rank-and-file Republicans. The GOP threat also changed voting behavior: it mobilized Democrats to assign greater importance to the ACA in their candidate selection and depressed the intent of Republicans to cast a vote based on health reform. In other words, the strategy of the Washington GOP backfired: repeal rallied Democrats to become more politically engaged and muted opposition among everyday Republicans.

Third, the ACA is giving rise to new constituents who rely on its benefits and share intense attachments to them. The GOP's repeal threat awoke several groups of beneficiaries, making them more fully appreciative of the new health care benefits by the 2018 elections than they were previously. Americans who had realized that the ACA expanded access before the 2016 elections became more supportive afterward. More striking, the GOP threat stirred greater appreciation for the ACA's impact among individuals who had not registered such views previously as well as among low-income people who were especially dependent on the new coverage (Zhu, Mettler, and Jacobs 2019).

New policy that creates new constituents represents a politically potent form of policy feedback (Campbell 2003). The ACA's decade of operations is now starting to coalesce new beneficiaries as a self-conscious set of constituents, although the extent to which political leaders or groups will mobilize them as such remains to be seen.

A fourth feature of the new politics of health reform is the ACA's impact on political efficacy (Mettler, Jacobs, and Zhu 2019). According to our panel data, between the ACA's passage in 2010 and the 2018 elections, the survival of health reform and distribution of its concrete benefits prodded individuals to higher levels of confidence in their individual competence to participate effectively in politics and lifted their confidence that government will respond. These effects hold up despite potent controls for political ideology, demographic factors, and other potential influences.

ACA Politics

During the ACA's first decade, it endured criticism from both the Left and the Right. While the two sides differed on their favored remedy, both shared a view of reform as a fixed endpoint instead of a process of evolution over time. This stagnant view blinded conservatives to the network of support for the ACA that now extends well beyond beneficiaries themselves to the well-organized ranks of medical providers, commercial insurers, pharmaceutical companies, and states that have adopted Medicaid expansion.

The aspirational Left's failure to understand the implementation of health reform as a process has handicapped it from appreciating the program-expanding dynamics that the ACA has initiated, including the growing number of states that have adopted expanded Medicaid. Its operations both highlight shortcomings and identify tangible remedies for future reform, such as expanding subsidies to make premiums and deductibles more affordable. Perhaps most important, the ACA sets the terms for new reforms by framing health care as a right of citizenship instead of a privilege earned in the workplace and by legitimating the government's responsibility for health care coverage of the working population instead of deferring to employers or the individual acting alone (Jacobs 2014).

Treating the ACA as an endpoint instead of a policy undergoing a process of development over time has also distorted judgments about its distributional effects—its winners and losers. While verdicts issued soon after the law's enactment may have been accurate at the time, they miss the changes that have ensued, including the "comebacks"—the groups of Americans who were initially considered to be on the losing end but are now benefiting. The Supreme Court's 2012 decision altered the original legislative plan by replacing the relatively straightforward national implementation of the new Medicaid benefits with cumbersome, uneven battles within each state. This created gruesome disparities in mortality and illness across states that adopted or failed to adopt the Medicaid expansion. As time has passed, however, the ranks of adopting states have steadily grown to 37, with 3 states in the process of accepting the new programs and more still in the process of debating it. States and groups of people who were initially declared "losers" are now coming back and gaining needed medical care; little attention has been given to these comebacks that resulted from the evolving process of reform.

There may also be signs that the initially anointed "winners" among powerful businesses and interests—such as pharmaceutical producers—are facing future constraints. As drug prices have continued to rise, there is rare bipartisan agreement on the problem and initial legislative steps toward a response, at least in the Senate. While significant concrete solutions are not imminent, the need to impose restraints on drug prices and the pharmaceutical industry now appears on the agendas of voters and federal and state governments.

The ACA also appears to be evolving from its early status as a politically vulnerable target amid Washington's partisan conflicts and gradually becoming a more politically resilient program than anticipated in the past. GOP politicians who attacked the ACA faced a backlash during the 2018 congressional elections, and the Republican governor of Kentucky, Matt Bevin, was punished for his attacks on the state's Medicaid program in the 2019 election. Compared to the electorate in the first four elections after the ACA was enacted, voters in 2018 who supported the ACA were intensely focused on the choice among candidates, had become more engaged politically than those who opposed health reform, and were more likely to take it into account when selecting candidates (Jacobs, Mettler, and Zhu 2019). While the ACA is not a "third rail of American politics" at this point, Republican politicians who attempt to repeal or roll it back now face scrutiny and potential political risks. Ambitious conservatives will have to take that into account in the future or face defeat.

Winston Churchill famously quipped in 1940, when British pilots fought off the German Luftwaffe and the threat of an invasion, that "never was so much owed by so many to so few." As the ACA emerges from a decade of fierce partisan warfare, its accomplishments also stand out: health reform has done so much but has been recognized for so little of it.

▪ ▪ ▪

Lawrence R. Jacobs is Walter F. and Joan Mondale Chair for Political Studies and director of the Center for the Study of Politics and Governance in the Hubert H. Humphrey School and the Department of Political Science at the University of Minnesota. He was awarded a visiting fellow position at All Souls College, Oxford University during 2019–20. Jacobs has published 16 books and edited volumes and dozens of articles on elections, legislative and presidential politics, elections and public opinion, and a range of public policies.
ljacobs@umn.edu

Suzanne Mettler is John L. Senior Professor of American Institutions in the Department of Government at Cornell University. She is the author of five books, most recently *The Government-Citizen Disconnect* (2018), which won the 2019 Alexander George Book Award of the International Society of Political Psychology. She was awarded a Guggenheim Fellowship and a Radcliffe Institute Fellowship in 2019.

References

Abramowitz, Alan I. 2010. *The Disappearing Center: Engaged Citizens, Polarization and American Democracy*. New Haven: Yale University Press.

Berry, Christopher R., Barry C. Burden, and William G. Howell. 2012. "The Lives and Deaths of Federal Programs, 1971–2003." In *Living Legislation: Durability, Change, and the Politics of American Lawmaking*, edited by Jeffery A. Jenkins and Eric M. Patashnik, 86–110. Chicago: University of Chicago Press.

Blumenthal, David, and James A. Morone. 2010. *The Heart of Power: Health and Politics in the Oval Office*. Berkeley: University of California Press.

Boyer, Peter J. 2010. "House Rule. Will John Boehner Control the Tea Party Congress?" *New Yorker*, The Political Scene, December 6. www.newyorker.com/magazine/2010/12/13/house-rule-peter-j-boyer.

Callaghan, Timothy, and Lawrence R. Jacobs. 2014. "Process Learning and the Implementation of Medicaid Reform." *Publius* 44, no. 4: 541–63.

Callaghan, Timothy, and Lawrence R. Jacobs. 2016. "Interest Group Conflict over Medicaid Expansion: The Surprising Impact of Public Advocates." *American Journal of Public Health* 106, no. 2: 308–13.

Callaghan, Timothy, and Lawrence R. Jacobs. 2017. "The Future of Health Care Reform: What Is Driving Enrollment?" *Journal of Health Politics, Policy and Law* 42, no. 2: 215–46.

Campbell, Andrea Louise. 2003. *How Policies Make Citizens: Senior Political Activism and the American Welfare State*. Princeton, NJ: Princeton University Press.

Edsall, Thomas. 2013. "The Obamacare Crisis." *New York Times*, November 19. www.nytimes.com/2013/11/20/opinion/edsall-the-obamacare-crisis.html.

Gilens, Martin, and Benjamin Page. 2014. "Testing Theories of American Politics: Elites, Interest Groups, and Average Citizens." *Perspectives on Politics* 12, no. 3: 564–81.

Hertel-Fernandez, Alexander, Theda Skocpol, and Daniel Lynch. 2016. "Business Associations, Conservative Networks, and the Ongoing Republican War over Medicaid Expansion." *Journal of Health Politics, Policy and Law* 41, no. 2: 239–86.

Holahan, John, and Linda Blumberg. 2017. "Instead of ACA Repeal and Replace, Fix It." Urban Institute, January. www.urban.org/sites/default/files/publication/87076/2001054-repeal-and-replace-aca-fix-it_2.pdf.

Jacobs, Lawrence. 2014. "Health Reform and the Future of American Politics." *Perspectives on Politics* 12, no. 3: 631–42.

Jacobs, Lawrence, and Joel Ario. 2012. "Post Election, the Affordable Care Act Leaves the Intensive Care Unit for Good." *Health Affairs* 31, no. 12: 2603–8.

Jacobs, Lawrence, and Timothy Callaghan. 2013. "Why States Expand Medicaid: Party, Resources, and History." *Journal of Health Politics, Policy and Law* 38, no. 5: 1023–50.

Jacobs, Lawrence, and Suzanne Mettler. 2018. "When and How New Policy Creates New Politics: Examining the Feedback Effects of the Affordable Care Act on Public Opinion." *Perspectives on Politics* 16, no. 2: 345–63.

Jacobs, Lawrence, Suzanne Mettler, and Ling Zhu. 2019. "Affordable Care Act Moving to New Stage of Public Acceptance." *Journal of Health Politics, Policy and Law* 44, no. 6: 911–17.

Jacobs, Lawrence, and Benjamin Page. 2005. "Who Influences U.S. Foreign Policy?" *American Political Science Review* 99, no. 1: 107–23.

Jacobs, Lawrence, and Theda Skocpol. 2015. *Health Care Reform and American Politics*. 3rd ed. New York: Oxford University Press.

Levendusky, Matthew. 2009. *The Partisan Sort: How Liberals Became Democrats and Conservatives Became Republicans*. Chicago, IL: University of Chicago Press.

Mettler, Suzanne. 2005. *Soldiers to Citizens: The G.I. Bill and the Making of the Greatest Generation*. New York: Oxford University Press.

Mettler, Suzanne. 2011. *The Submerged State: How Invisible Government Policies Undermine American Democracy*. Chicago: University of Chicago Press.

Mettler, Suzanne, Lawrence Jacobs, and Ling Zhu. 2019. "The Pathways of Policy Feedback: How Health Reform Influences Political Efficacy and Participation." Unpublished manuscript.

Miller, Sarah, Sean Altekruse, Norman Johnson, and Laura Wherry. 2019. "Medicaid and Mortality: New Evidence from Linked Survey and Administrative Data." NBER Working Paper No. 26081, National Bureau of Economic Research. www.nber.org/papers/w26081.

Patashnik, Eric M. 2008. *Reforms at Risk: What Happens after Major Policy Changes Are Enacted*. Princeton, NJ: Princeton University Press.

Skocpol, Theda, and Alexander Hertel-Fernandez. 2016. "The Koch Network and Republican Party Extremism." *Perspectives on Politics* 14: 681–99.

Taber, Charles S., and Milton Lodge. 2006. "Motivated Skepticism in the Evaluation of Political Beliefs." *American Journal of Political Science*. 50, no. 3: 755–69.

Tax Policy Center. 2018. "Key Elements of the US Tax System." Briefing Book. www.taxpolicycenter.org/briefing-book/what-tax-changes-did-affordable-care-act-make (accessed February 11, 2020).

Zhu, Ling, Suzanne Mettler, and Lawrence Jacobs. 2019. "How Policy Threat Influences Feedback Effects: The Public Backlash to Republican Efforts to Repeal Health Reform." Paper presented at the Annual Meeting of the American Political Science Association, Washington, DC, August 29–September 1.

The ACA a Decade In: Resilience, Impact, and Vulnerabilities

Mark A. Peterson
University of California Los Angeles

Abstract A decade after its enactment, the Affordable Care Act remains both politically viable and consequential, despite Republican efforts to end it. The law's impact on insurance coverage is substantial but remains distant from universal coverage, while its contributions to cost control are at best limited. National public opinion data collected by the author in 2018 reveal both strengths and vulnerabilities in the act.

Keywords Affordable Care Act, public opinion, insurance coverage, cost containment

Those familiar with the film *Apollo 13* will recall the scene. Having suffered a nearly disastrous explosion en route to the moon, and after a slingshot around it to return to Earth, the crew of the hobbled spacecraft had to execute a near perfect manual burn to set a viable course for Earth reentry. If they hit the atmosphere with too steep a trajectory, the capsule and crew would incinerate. Too shallow, they would bounce off the atmosphere and disappear into the oblivion of space. Given the fortunate ending, we know that they successfully navigated into what *Apollo 13* Commander Jim Lovell described as that "very narrow pie-shaped wedge."

Were Lovell a health policy historian, he could have been recounting the passage of the Affordable Care Act (ACA) in 2010. Numerous past health care reform initiatives had bounced off the governing system's unresponsive firmament, ignored, lost without a trace in the political ether. Other proposals, like Bill Clinton's Health Security Act, had slammed into an unforgiving political atmosphere, burning up and leaving damaging debris in their wakes. The ACA, however, found the path to enactment, the very

Journal of Health Politics, Policy and Law, Vol. 45, No. 4, August 2020
DOI 10.1215/03616878-8255517 © 2020 by Duke University Press

first reform legislation to secure floor votes in the House and Senate. Even in the best overall political-institutional context for enacting health care reform in US history, the pie-shaped wedge was truly narrow (Peterson 2019: chap. 11). Passage came in the Senate by overcoming a filibuster with no votes to spare. Final approval in the House rested on just a three-vote margin.

Legislative enactment is but a necessary, not sufficient, outcome. Achieve policy goals is the point. Not even designed to orbit the earth, Alan Shepard's first US manned space flight in 1961 may have seemed intended to do nothing more than thrust a live American into weightlessness and return him alive and unharmed to the ground, but even that mission was part of an orchestrated plan to fulfill national objectives framed by the Cold War competition with the Soviet Union and eventual advances in science. The ACA's political success, however thrilling given its uniqueness, would have meaning only if it had a demonstrable positive impact on the health care system. As with all health care reform initiatives, its two most prominent objectives were to expand substantially insurance coverage and to do something meaningful to rein in rising health care costs, joined by features aimed to promote higher-quality care, invigorate the health professions, and advance population health (Kaiser Family Foundation 2010). At the 10–year mark since its passage, assessment of the ACA confronts three core questions. First, did the law really survive intact its fiery plunge through the intensely partisan and resistant political atmosphere of contemporary America? Second, how well has it fulfilled the promise to enlarge markedly the ranks of the insured population and set a course for universal coverage? Third, how effectively has it put in place mechanisms to contain growing health care expenditures—overall, for government budgets and taxpayers, and out-of-pocket for individuals and families.

The answers in all three respects are mixed. In part that reflects positive returns. The ACA has revealed perhaps surprising resilience, put insurance cards into the hands of millions previously outside the system, and even contributed to some degree of reduced financial burdens. At the same time, all of these gains have been incomplete, remain vulnerable, and are threatened by underlying forces in the political economy. The path to a more secure future for either the ACA or a more ambitious successor is far from clear.

Political Resilience

In the history of American social benefit programs, the ACA has proven to be one of the most susceptible to disruption and outright repeal, risking joining the Medicare Catastrophic Coverage Act of 1989 on the ash heap of domestic policy (Peterson 2018b). A social policy program that cannot manage to stay in the statute books is not one of consequence. The enactment of the ACA on those meager entirely party-line margins arguably did much to fuel the Tea Party mobilization on the right. That in turn helped enable the 2010 midterm electoral wave that allowed Republicans not only to recapture the majority in the House of Representatives but also to assume a commanding position in the states—state legislatures flipped from 54% Democratic control to 52% in Republican hands, governorships went from 52% blue to 58% red, and the GOP gained the trifecta of unified government in 40% of the states.[1] While the new Republican House majority immediately launched repeated efforts to repeal or eviscerate Obamacare, their fellow partisans in the states initiated collective lawsuits against it and blocked the Medicaid expansions that had been made voluntary by the US Supreme Court's ruling in *NFIB v. Sebelius* (567 U.S. 519 [2012]).

For much of 10 years since the statute's enactment, its political health looked precarious. It decidedly lacked the popular acclaim of the sort that arose to undergird programs like Social Security and Medicare. The Kaiser Family Foundation has fielded monthly national tracking polls throughout this period, including fairly regularly taking the temperature of the ACA in the body politic by asking the question: "As you may know, a health reform bill was signed into law in 2010. Given what you know about the health reform law, do you have a generally favorable or generally unfavorable opinion of it?" (Kaiser Family Foundation 2019b). Although health care reform in general and even President Obama's proposed plan had enjoyed net support of 30 percentage points and higher, in the month after formal passage the ACA mustered a positive view from only 46% of the respondents, disfavor from 40%, and a "don't know" opinion from 14%. Late the following year the ACA was held in particularly low regard, with only one-third supportive and just over half now disapproving. Later still, from February 2013 to November 2014 those with a favorable view stayed in the 30% range, including in the low 30% range following the disastrous rollout of HealthCare.gov, the federal website for enrolling in the newly available market exchange plans. For a substantial part of the last decade the law was underwater in public opinion.

Three interrelated events saved the ACA from this unstable purgatory. First, ongoing Democratic control of the Senate until 2015 and President

---

1. These data were assembled from various election results reported at ballotpedia.org and the National Conference of State Legislatures (ncsl.org).

Barack Obama's reelection to a second term lasting through 2016 meant that Republican efforts at repeal could not succeed until at least 3 years after the full implementation of the ACA's coverage benefits and preexisting condition protections. Consistent with the positive policy-feedback literature and unlike the case with the Medicare Catastrophic Coverage Act, that was sufficient time to anchor the program in the public's expectations and the interests of such stakeholders as insurers, hospitals, and other providers (Peterson 2018b).

Second, the explicit Republican campaign in 2017 to abolish the law—the principal legislative activity of the year, at least until the passage of the Tax Cuts and Jobs Act in December—accorded the public every reason to pay attention to the coverage expansions and protections afforded by the ACA and rise in their defense. Congressional Budget Office (2017) scoring of the Republican plans, which went beyond repeal to curtailing long-standing Medicaid coverage, revealed that 23 million people would lose insurance. More would be uninsured than before the ACA's enactment. Preexisting condition protections would also be largely undone. At the time of the 2016 election, in the Kaiser Family Foundation survey the public's views of the ACA split 43% favorable and 45% unfavorable. Soon after Senator John McCain famously gave the thumbs down to the Senate version of repeal and replace in July 2017, helping defeat it, public support had turned favorable at 52% to 39%. Tracking the same respondents through five waves in a panel study from 2010 to 2018, Jacobs, Mettler, and Zhu (2019: 913) also show a marked increase in support for the law.

In 2018 Darin DeWitt and I designed a health care policy and politics module for that year's Cooperative Congressional Election Study (CCES), a national survey of public attitudes built around common content and the specific investigations of 60 research teams (Ansolabehere, Schaffner, and Luks 2019; Peterson 2018a). Each team's module is administered to a nationally representative sample of about 1,000 respondents. We asked about a large number of specific provisions in health care legislation, without identifying which were associated with the ACA and which derived from the Republican proposals. Of the eight that tracked with actual features of the ACA, despite the ambiguity about the law as a whole, all drew supermajorities of public support, ranging from 60% to 80% (mean, 69.4%). Even the most redistributive and likely to be especially contentious—having Medicaid cover all low-income uninsured adults and providing subsidies to Americans of modest means to buy private insurance—garnered endorsement from over 60% of the respondents.

Third, beyond advocating dismantling the ACA, Republicans weakened their political standing even further by offering replacement approaches that alienated the public and influential interests. When we asked respondents in the 2018 CCES whether they had a generally favorable or unfavorable opinion of the Republican proposals, among the 80% who expressed an opinion, only one-third were supportive and two-thirds opposed. Of the five provisions in our survey associated with the 2017 Republican plans, public support averaged 39.6%. The only one to attract majority support would allow insurers to sell plans that traded lower premiums for higher out-of-pocket costs and uncovered services. At the same time, though, 65.6% of our sample favored a provision that would "require insurers in the individual and small group health insurance markets to cover" the list of 10 "essential benefits" formally included in the ACA, which only 13.1% opposed. With respect to Medicaid, only 35.5% supported denying coverage to able-bodied adults and fewer still (28.1%) agreed with capped federal financial allocations to the states joined with greater state flexibility to determine whom and what to cover. The Republican's legislative efforts also antagonized almost the entire domain of stakeholder interests, many of which had been that party's past allies in health care reform debates. The final GOP initiative of 2017, drafted by Republican Senators Lindsay Graham (SC) and Bill Cassidy (LA), was publicly endorsed by just five conservative groups and opposed by 114 organizations, including most of the provider community and the health insurance industry (Bajaj and Thompson 2017; Zernike, Abelson, and Goodnough 2017).

Opponents to the ACA have nonetheless been able to weaken the ACA and perhaps set the stage for its ultimate downfall. The Trump administration has taken a number of executive actions that have lessened its coverage and protections, leading, among other things, to a couple million people joining the uninsured population (Galewitz 2019). The Tax Cuts and Jobs Act of 2017 did not formally terminate the individual mandate to have insurance coverage, but it did zero out the associated penalty administered through the tax collection system (Jost 2017). That, in turn, has provided a foundation for the statutory interpretation claim, in *Texas v. United States* pursued by 20 Republican state attorneys general and accepted by a federal district court judge in Texas, that the rest of the law depends on the mandate and thus must be declared invalid. The case will be decided by the US Supreme Court (Keith 2019).

Considering the public confusion about what the ACA includes and does, the extreme partisan polarization surrounding the law, the dramatic shifts in the nation's electoral winds at both the national and state level, the myriad court challenges and resistance to full implementation in many of the states, and every effort of President Trump's administration to use executive actions to debilitate one of his predecessor's primary legislative achievements, it may be surprising that the ACA remains viable and functioning 10 years out. When NASA's Houston Control scrambled to save the *Apollo 13* crew, striving through creative adaptation to keep the astronauts alive and give them a shot at a safe return, the motivating dictum was "failure is not an option" (SpaceActs, n.d.). Given what the Congressional Budget Office and other analysts calculated would be the consequence of the ACA's demise, perhaps it applies equally in this case.

The ACA's Impact on Insurance Coverage

The primary mission of the ACA was to make substantial progress toward addressing the outlier status of the United States as the world's sole democracy and developed economy that did not reach anything proximate to universal health care coverage. The estimated consequences of repeal—the millions who would be kicked off the insurance roles—suggest that the progress toward that objective was substantial. A variety of metrics can be used to capture the size of the uninsured population—for example, at the time queried, for some portion of the year, and for longer than a year—and by all of them the implementation of the new health care law had fairly quick and significant effects. The National Health Interview Survey revealed that in 2015, halfway toward this 10–year anniversary, those with an episode of being uninsured during some period in the year fell from 24.4% to 18.1%, and the long-term uninsured dropped from 15.7% to just 9.1% (Cohen, Martinez, and Zammitti 2016). Moreover, the percentage uninsured dropped by a third to a half for every demographic group, from those that had the highest rates when the ACA was enacted (e.g., Hispanics and young adults) to those already at the low end (e.g., children and whites overall) (Garrett and Gangopadhyaya 2016). After 2015 the uninsured percentage continued to fall, reaching the lowest points in 2016–17, with the population-wide figure below 8%. Then came subsequent increases, returning to 8.5% overall, or 27.5 million individuals (Keith 2019). Not only is that a reversal, but even the moment of glory in 2016 was a far cry from the international standard of universal coverage.

The previous singular effort to expand insurance coverage came in 1965 with the enactment of Medicare and Medicaid. I estimate that, with about half the elderly and measurably few of the poor having either private or public benefits of any kind before their enactment, by 1975 the two programs had brought coverage to about 35 million Americans who would otherwise have been entirely uninsured, roughly 16% of the nation's population (Kaiser Family Foundation 2013; Mikulic 2019; Moon 1996). In 2010, that was the natural limit of what even a truly universal program could accomplish. "Only" 16% of the population—about 49 million people—were still uninsured. The ACA by 2016 cut that percentage roughly in half. That may seem less consequential than Medicare and Medicaid, but it is important to keep two other factors in mind. First, the services covered and financial protections provided by Medicare and Medicaid fell far short of today's typical employer-sponsored plans, inclusive of additional ACA provisions like prohibitions on annual or lifetime caps, free preventive services, or the 10 essential benefits required of ACA exchange plans. Second, Medicare's restriction to one age group and Medicaid's coverage of only certain categories of the poor meant that they, unlike the 2010 law, did not create even a potential pathway to universal coverage, if only for US citizens and lawful permanent residents.

Going forward, however, there are at least three fundamental threats to what the ACA has accomplished in coverage. One reflects the fact that possession of an insurance card does not mean that one is well insured and without barriers to needed health care services. The ACA has done nothing to reduce the aggregate percentage of what the Commonwealth Fund identifies as the "underinsured"—those facing out-of-pocket costs so significant that they lead to foregoing primary or specialist medical care, missing treatments, or not filling prescriptions. The 2018 aggregate figure of 45% for adults 19–64 years old was unchanged from 2010 (Collins, Bhupal, and Doty 2019).

The other two are inherent in the structure of the ACA itself. To avoid major political roadblocks, the architecture of the law—unlike past comprehensive reform plans from President Truman to President Clinton—is predicated on minimizing disruptions in the existing system (Peterson 2019: chap. 11). It keeps largely intact employer-sponsored insurance, Medicare, and Medicaid and builds on them to expand coverage. Cracks in those underpinnings to the insurance system could undermine the ACA coverage model. The ongoing financial viability of employer-sponsored insurance for both employers and employees, for example, might well be questioned. As of 2018 the mean total annual premium for a single employee in the United States came close to $8,000; for family coverage it was just shy of $20,000. On average, the employee premium contribution and deductible hit 11.5% of median household income (Collins, Radley, and Baumgartner 2019).

The public perceives that there is a broad set of risks to the system. In our 2018 CCES survey, we asked the respondents whether seven changes occurring in the realm of employment and insurance, such as contracting out jobs, would result in "certain failure" of employer-sponsored insurance, pose a "threat" to it, or not be a problem. Individually the "certain failure" responses fell below a third, but in total 60% selected that category for at least one of the seven factors. In the meantime, the current Medicare program and its financial stability remain caught in the maw of the nation's polarized politics, while the eligible population grows dramatically with the aging of the baby boom generation (Aaron and Lambrew 2008).

The ACA has one other feature, compelled by contemporary political forces, that stands in the way of ever achieving universal coverage. It explicitly prohibits the inclusion of undocumented immigrants, which in 2017 the Pew Research Center estimated to be 10.5 million individuals or roughly 4 in 10 of the currently uninsured (Passel 2019). In our 2018 CCES survey, there was strong opposition—58.9% to 22.2%—to "allow[ing] undocumented immigrants to receive financial help from the government to buy health insurance," much less be given access to direct benefit programs like Medicaid.

The ACA's Impact on Health Care Costs

The ACA also had the stated mission of tackling the high cost of health care in the United States. As President Obama himself put it in his September 2009 health care speech to a joint session of Congress,

> There is the problem of rising costs. We spend one-and-a-half times more per person on health care than any other country, but we aren't any healthier for it. . . . Our health care system is placing an unsustainable burden on taxpayers. When health care costs grow at the rate they have, it puts greater pressure on programs like Medicare and Medicaid. . . . Put simply, our health care problem is our deficit problem. Nothing else even comes close.

Pass his health care reform initiative, he pronounced, and "it will slow the growth of health care costs for our families, our businesses, and our government" (Obama 2009). The president's senior advisers and a number of allies in the analytical community often repeated various versions of the refrain that provisions in the law would "bend the cost curve" (e.g., Orszag and Emanuel 2010: 602). Campaigning for the presidency, candidate Obama projected that his health care plan would "cut the cost of a typical family's premiums by $2,500" (best understood in relation to what premiums would otherwise be) (Kessler 2012).

The problem is that the law was simply devoid of the kind of cost-control mechanisms, from budgets to rate setting, that had proven effective abroad or in some states and were included in some form in previous reform proposals like President Bill Clinton's Health Security Act (Peterson 2019: chaps. 4, 10). Because every dollar of expenditure is a dollar of income for someone in the system, aggressive restraints on spending would seriously pinch influential stakeholders whose political support was needed (Evans 1997). In addition, what most voters worry about is what they pay out of pocket, rather than system totals (Blendon et al. 2006). The drafters of the ACA turned to less empirically proven but conceptually attractive devices to lower costs through the more hidden-hand approach of enhanced efficiency, such as incentives, deterrents, and competition; and a more effective delivery system, such as through coordination of care and investments in innovation (Oberlander 2011; White 2018). Oberlander (2011) aptly captured the experimental and scattershot methods in the ACA as "throwing darts," looking with more optimism than conviction to see which ones might actually land on the target and score (see also Marmor, Oberlander, and White 2009).

Right from the start many specialists in the health policy field, especially those with eyes on the comparative experience, did not expect this eclectic collection of technical remedies, disincentives, funding streams, and demonstration projects to have much sway on the costs borne by any of the payers in the health care system (Gusmano 2011; Marmor, Oberlander, and White 2009; Oberlander 2011; White 2018). The intervention with likely the farthest-reaching impact—the so-called Cadillac tax that was claimed, with considerable controversy, to discourage excessively generous employer-sponsored insurance plans—was set to begin fully 8 years after enactment of the law (2018), then was delayed by congressional action until 2022, and now is at risk of repeal (in July 2019 the US House of Representatives voted 419–6 to kill it) (Gusmano 2011; Luthi 2019; Oberlander 2011; White 2018). The only other provision that had some real regulatory teeth and might have been consequential for at least its target of Medicare spending, the Independent Payment Advisory Board and its implementation tools, was never allowed to become operational before it was terminated by Public Law No. 115–123, the Bipartisan Budget Act of 2018, (Oberlander and Spivack 2018).

That is not to say that passage of the ACA had demonstrably no bearing on the costs of health care. In the years immediately following enactment, there appeared to be a slowing down in medical inflation and reduced rates of growth in per capita national health expenditures, private health insurance premiums, and Medicare and Medicaid spending (Hartman et al. 2018; Peterson 2019: chap. 11). By some estimates, "total health care costs were almost $650 billion less than anticipated" in pre-ACA 2010 projections (Glickman, DiMagno, and Emanuel 2019: 1151). It is difficult, however, to disentangle the lingering effects of the Great Recession of 2008–9, the influence of the ACA, and the role of other dynamics in the health care system (Blumenthal, Stremikis, and Cutler 2013; White 2018). Moreover, the system-wide metrics of swelling costs since full implementation of the law in 2013 show some signs of returning to the earlier patterns (Peterson 2019: chap. 11; Sisko et al. 2019). Premiums and deductibles for employer-sponsored coverage have climbed as well as in recent years, well over growth rates in median income, and include shifting burdens to workers' wallets (Collins, Radley, and Baumgartner 2019; Kaiser Family Foundation 2019a). As desired by the Obama admin-istration, health care system features like electronic health records and accountable care organizations have soared. For electronic health records, just under half of physician offices used them in 2010, compared to nearly 9 in 10 in 2017, and accountable care organizations have leapt from 58 in 2011 to 1,011 in 2018, about half involving Medicare and Medicaid (Muhlestein et al. 2018; Office of National Coordinator for Health Infor-mation Technology 2017). Over a third of health care payments in that latest year fit with value-based payment models (Lagasse 2018). And yet all of that modernization of the US health care system has come without clear or consistent beneficial financial effects (e.g., Schultze and Fry 2019). One area where one can have some confidence is that the Medicaid expansion feature of the ACA mitigated to some extent financial burdens on the poor and diminished the previous regressivity of American health care financing (Jacobs and Selden 2019; McKenna, Alcala, and Grande 2018).

Conclusion

Passage of the ACA 10 years ago depended on setting a precise political course with little margin for error. The calculations that made that possible instilled the law with greater political resiliency than might have been imagined at the time, but also assured that its mission to drive toward universal coverage and constrain health care expenditures, including at the level of families and individuals, would produce mixed results at best and be weighted toward coverage expansions rather than cost control. The

Republican Party of the twenty-first century, in full display during the repeal efforts of the 115th Congress (2017–18), has abandoned the commitments of some past leaders to expanded insurance and comprehensive access to medical care—themes promoted in the 1970s and 1990s by President Richard Nixon, Senate Republican Leader Robert Dole, and Senators John Chafee and Jim Jeffords—focusing instead on promoting health plans with lower premiums but limited benefits, private market competition, and restricted federal spending (Peterson 2019: chap. 12). With the impossibility of serious Republican partners and the inherent shortcomings of the ACA architecture to address coverage and costs, Democrats entered the 2020 election season—the law's tenth birthday—debating whether the ACA offered a viable foundation for a substantially more expansive next step or whether it was necessary to hearken back to President Truman and the party's original pledge of tax-payer-financed national health insurance under the current rubric of "Medicare for All." If it is the latter, will such an initiative hit the political atmosphere too directly, burning up on entry and thwarting capture of the White House in the next presidential election? Or will it skip off a resistant atmosphere, summarily rejected like most past reform efforts? Or will it pass through, dented, singed, and missing some pieces, but landing functional on the health policy terrain? Those will be the central questions of the next decade in health care reform.

▪ ▪ ▪

Mark A. Peterson is professor of public policy, political science, and law and former chair of the Department of Public Policy at the UCLA Luskin School of Public Affairs. A specialist on American national government and the policy process, he is an elected member of the National Academy of Social Insurance, past recipient of a Robert Wood Johnson Foundation Investigator Award in Health Policy Research, and former editor of *JHPPL*. His book manuscript, "American Sisyphus: Health Care and the Challenge of Transformative Policymaking," is a comprehensive study of the nation's century of health care reform politics.
markap@ucla.edu

References

Aaron, Henry J., and Jeanne M. Lambrew. 2008. *Reforming Medicare: Options, Tradeoffs, and Opportunities.* Washington, DC: Brookings Institution Press.

Ansolabehere, Stephen, Brian Schaffner, and Sam Luks. 2019. "Guide to the 2018 Cooperative Congressional Election Study." Harvard Dataverse, v. 6. doi.org/10.7910 /DVN/ZSBZ7K/WZWCZ1.

Bajaj, Vikas, and Stuart Thompson. 2017. "Republicans Are Remarkably Good at Uniting Opposition against Themselves." *New York Times*, September 25.

Blendon, Robert J., Kelly Hunt, John M. Benson, Channtal Fleischerfresser, and Tami Buhr. 2006. "Understanding the American Public's Health Priorities: A 2006 Perspective." *Health Affairs* 25, suppl. 1: w508–15. doi.org/10.1377/hlthaff.25.w508.

Blumenthal, David, Kristof Stremikis, and David Cutler. 2013. "Health Care Spending—A Giant Slain or Sleeping?" *New England Journal of Medicine* 369, no. 26: 2551–57.

CBO (Congressional Budget Office). 2017. "H.R. 1628, American Health Care Act of 2017." www.cbo.gov/system/files/115th-congress-2017–2018/costestimate/hr1628 aspassed.pdf.

Cohen, Robin A., Michael E. Martinez, and Emily P. Zammitti. 2016. "Health Insurance Coverage: Early Release of Estimates from the National Health Interview Survey, 2015." US Department of Health and Human Services, Centers for Disease Control and Prevention, National Center for Health Statistics, May. www .cdc.gov/nchs/data/nhis/earlyrelease/insur201605.pdf.

Collins, Sara R., Herman K. Bhupal, and Michelle M. Doty. 2019. "Health Insurance Coverage Eight Years after the ACA: Fewer Uninsured Americans and Shorter Coverage Gaps, but More Underinsured." Commonwealth Fund, February. www .commonwealthfund.org/sites/default/files/2019-08/Collins_hlt_ins_coverage_8_ years_after_ACA_2018_biennial_survey_sb_v2.pdf.

Collins, Sara R., David C. Radley, and Jesse C. Baumgartner. 2019. "Trends in Employer Health Care Coverage, 2008–2018: Higher Costs for Workers and Their Families." Commonwealth Fund, November. www.commonwealthfund.org/sites /default/files/2019-11/Collins_state_premium_trends_2008_2018_db_1.pdf.

Evans, Robert G. 1997. "Going for the Gold: The Redistributive Agenda behind Market-Based Health Care Reform." *Journal of Health Politics, Policy and Law* 22, no. 2: 427–65.

Galewitz, Phil. 2019. "Breaking a Ten-Year Streak, the Number of Uninsured Americans Rises." *Kaiser Health News*, September 10. khn.org/news/number-of -americans-without-insurance-rises-in-2018/.

Garrett, Bowen, and Anuj Gangopadhyaya. 2016. "Who Gained Health Insurance Coverage under the ACA, and Where Do They Live?" Robert Wood Johnson Foundation and Urban Institute, December. www.urban.org/sites/default/files /publication/86761/2001041-who-gained-health-insurance-coverage-under-the-aca -and-where-do-they-live.pdf.

Glickman, Aaron, Sarah S. P. DiMagno, and Ezekiel J. Emanuel. 2019. "Next Phase in Effective Cost Control in Health Care." *JAMA* 321, no. 12: 1151–52.

Gusmano, Michael K. 2011. "Do We Really Want to Control Health Care Spending?" *Journal of Health Politics, Policy and Law* 36, no. 3: 495–500.

Hartman, Micah, Anne B. Martin, Nathan Espinosa, Aaron Catlin, and the National Health Expenditure Accounts Team. 2018. "National Health Care Spending in

2016: Spending and Enrollment Growth Slow after Initial Coverage Expansions."
Health Affairs 37, no. 1: 150–60.

Jacobs, Lawrence R., Suzanne Mettler, and Ling Zhu. 2019. "Affordable Care Act
Moving to New Stage of Public Acceptance." *Journal of Health Politics, Policy
and Law* 44, no. 6: 911–16.

Jacobs, Paul D., and Thomas M. Selden. 2019. "Changes in the Equity of U.S. Health
Care Financing in the Period 2005–16." *Health Affairs* 38, no. 11: 1791–1800.

Jost, Timothy. 2017. "The Tax Bill and the Individual Mandate: What Happened, and
What Does It Mean?" *Health Affairs Blog*, December 20. doi.org/10.1377/
hblog20171220.323429.

Kaiser Family Foundation. 2010. "Summary of New Health Reform Law." March 26.
www.kff.org/health-reform/fact-sheet/summary-of-the-affordable-care-act/.

Kaiser Family Foundation. 2013. "Medicare Enrollment, 1966–2013." July 15. www
.kff.org/medicare/slide/medicare-enrollment-1966–2013/.

Kaiser Family Foundation. 2019a. "Employer Health Benefits: 2019 Annual Survey."
September. files.kff.org/attachment/Report-Employer-Health-Benefits-Annual
-Survey-2019.

Kaiser Family Foundation. 2019b. "KFF Health Tracking Poll: The Public's Views on
the ACA." October 15. www.kff.org/interactive/kff-health-tracking-poll-the-publics
-views-on-the-aca/#?response=Favorable—Unfavorable&aRange=all.

Keith, Katie. 2019. "Texas Arguments Lead Heavy ACA Action." *Health Affairs* 38,
no. 10: 1614–15.

Kessler, Glenn. 2012. "Romney's Whopper Claim on an Obama Health Care Pledge."
Washington Post, July 3. www.washingtonpost.com/blogs/fact-checker/post/romneys
-whopper-claim-on-an-obama-health-care-pledge/2012/07/03/gJQAVhk3IW_blog
.html.

Lagasse, Jeff. 2018. "Healthcare Payments Tied to Value-Based Care on the Rise, Now
at 34 Percent." *Healthcare IT News*, October 24. www.healthcarefinancenews.com
/news/healthcare-payments-tied-value-based-care-rise-now-34-percent.

Luthi, Susannah. 2019. "House Votes to Repeal Obamacare's 'Cadillac Tax.'" *Modern
Healthcare*, July 17. www.modernhealthcare.com/government/house-votes-repeal
-obamacares-cadillac-tax.

Marmor, Theodore, Jonathan Oberlander, and Joseph White. 2009. "The Obama
Administration's Options for Health Care Cost Control: Hope versus Reality."
Annals of Internal Medicine 150, no. 7: 485–89.

McKenna, Ryan M., Hector E. Alcala, and David T. Grande. 2018. "The Affordable
Care Act Attenuates Financial Strain According to Poverty Level." *Inquiry* 55, no. 1:
1–14.

Mikulic, Matej. 2019. "Total Medicaid Enrollment from 1966 to 2018." *Statista*, August
9. www.statista.com/statistics/245347/total-medicaid-enrollment-since-1966/.

Moon, Marilyn. 1996. *Medicare Now and in the Future*. 2nd ed. Washington, DC:
Urban Institute.

Muhlestein, David, Robert S. Saunders, Robert Richards, and Mark B. McClellan.
2018. "Recent Progress in the Value Journey: Growth of ACOs and Value-Based

Payment Models in 2018." *Health Affairs Blog*, August 14. www.healthaffairs.org /do/10.1377/hblog20180810.481968/full/.

Obama, Barack. 2009. "Obama's Health Care Speech to Congress." *New York Times*, September 9.

Oberlander, Jonathan. 2011. "Throwing Darts: Americans' Elusive Search for Health Care Cost Control." *Journal of Health Politics, Policy and Law* 36, no. 3: 477–84.

Oberlander, Jonathan, and Steven B. Spivack. 2018. "Technocratic Dreams, Political Realities: The Rise and Demise of Medicare's Independent Payment Advisory Board." *Journal of Health Politics, Policy and Law* 43, no. 3: 483–510.

Office of the National Coordinator for Health Information Technology. 2017. "Office-Based Physician Electronic Health Record Adoption." Health HIT Dashboard. dashboard.healthit.gov/quickstats/pages/physician-ehr-adoption-trends.php (accessed February 11, 2020).

Orszag, Peter R., and Ezekiel J. Emanuel. 2010. "Health Care Reform and Cost Control." *New England Journal of Medicine* 363: 601–3.

Passel, Jeffrey S. 2019. "Measuring Illegal Immigration: How Pew Research Center Counts Unauthorized Immigrants in the U.S." FactTank, July 12. www.pew research.org/fact-tank/2019/07/12/how-pew-research-center-counts-unauthorized -immigrants-in-us/.

Peterson, Mark A. 2018a. Cooperative Congressional Election Study (CCES). cces .gov.harvard.edu (accessed April 20, 2020).

Peterson, Mark A. 2018b. "Reversing Course on Obamacare: Why Not Another Medicare Catastrophic?" *Journal of Health Politics, Policy and Law* 43, no. 4: 605–50.

Peterson, Mark A. 2019. "American Sisyphus: Health Care and the Challenge of Transformative Policymaking." Unpublished manuscript.

Schultze, Fred, and Erika Fry. 2019. "Death by 1,000 Clicks: Where Electronic Health Records Went Wrong." *Kaiser Health News*, March 18. khn.org/news/death-by-a -thousand-clicks/.

Sisko, Andrea M., Sean P. Keehan, John A. Poisal, Gigi A. Cuckler, Sheila D. Smith, Andrew J. Madison, Kathryn E. Rennie, and James C. Hardesty. 2019. "National Health Expenditures Projections, 2018–27: Economic and Demographic Trends Drive Spending and Enrollment Growth." *Health Affairs* 38, no. 3: 491–501.

SpaceActs.com. n.d. "Origin of Apollo 13 Quote: 'Failure Is Not an Option.'" www .spaceacts.com/notanoption.htm (accessed November 26, 2019).

White, Joseph. 2018. "Hypotheses and Hope: Policy Analysis and Cost Controls (or Not) in the Affordable Care Act." *Journal of Health Politics, Policy and Law* 43, no. 3: 455–82.

Zernike, Kate, Reed Abelson, and Abby Goodnough. 2017. "New Effort to Kill Obamacare Is Called 'the Most Radical.'" *New York Times*, September 21. www .nytimes.com/2017/09/21/health/graham-cassidy-obamacare-repeal-.html.

Race, Policy Feedbacks, and Political Resilience

The Affordable Care Act's Enduring Resilience

Larry Levitt
Kaiser Family Foundation

Abstract The Affordable Care Act (ACA) has taken numerous blows, both from the courts and from opponents seeking to undermine it. Yet, due to its policy design and the political forces the ACA has unleashed, the law has shown remarkable resilience. While there remain ongoing efforts to undo the ACA, the smart money has to be on its continued existence.

Keywords Affordable Care Act, health reform, politics

Following the 2016 election, I was quoted in the *Washington Post* as saying the Affordable Care Act (ACA) "as we know it would seem to be toast" (Goldstein 2016). Though the ACA has indeed been altered by the Trump administration and Congress since that election, this quote turned out to be a bit of an overstatement. The ACA is certainly still alive and has shown remarkable resilience since its enactment, reflecting its policy design, changes made legislatively and by the courts, and the politics surrounding it.

The 2012 Supreme Court Decision

The first hit the ACA took was the 2012 Supreme Court decision in *NFIB et al v. Sebelius*. In that decision, the court upheld the constitutionality of the law's individual mandate but ruled that the expansion of Medicaid to all individuals with incomes up to 138% of the federal poverty level would have to be voluntary for states (US Supreme Court 2012). This decision significantly changed the course of the ACA. Currently, 14 states have not

Journal of Health Politics, Policy and Law, Vol. 45, No. 4, August 2020
DOI 10.1215/03616878-8255529   © 2020 by Duke University Press

adopted the Medicaid expansion—even though the federal government will pay 90% of the cost—leaving many people below poverty in those states with no affordable health coverage (KFF 2019d).

The ACA has certainly been less effective at increasing health insurance coverage without all states expanding Medicaid. However, many blue states as well as red states have chosen to expand Medicaid, often with federal waivers such as work requirements to put a more conservative imprint on expansion. It is hard to say for sure what effect the Court's decision has had on the politics of the ACA. On the one hand, if all states had been required to expand Medicaid, it might have built an even bigger and stronger constituency for the law. On the other hand, it is quite possible that requiring recalcitrant states to expand would have generated an even stronger backlash against the ACA and made it less politically sustainable. Giving states a choice over whether to expand Medicaid means that those that make that choice may in the end be more invested in the law. This played out during the 2017 effort to repeal and replace the ACA, including rolling back the Medicaid expansion, when a number of Republican governors who had expanded Medicaid weighed in against repeal.

Large Premium Increases and Insurer Exits

In the first few years of the ACA's full implementation starting in 2014, premiums in the Health Insurance Marketplace were generally lower than expected (Levitt, Cox, and Claxton 2016). However, it turned out that premiums were too low, as insurers misestimated costs, particularly related to the relative shares of enrollees with and without preexisting conditions, and many insurers lost money in the Marketplace as a result (Levitt, Cox, and Claxton 2017). This produced a significant market adjustment, as insurers raised premiums substantially and many exited the ACA Marketplace and the individual market generally going into 2017. The average benchmark premium increased by 20% nationally for 2017 (KFF 2019b), and the share of Marketplace enrollees with a choice of only one insurer increased from 2% in 2016 to 21% in 2017 (Fehr, Kamal, and Cox 2019).

The ACA seemed on the ropes, but the structure of the law's premium subsidies has promoted stability in the market, making it resilient to premium increases. The framers of the ACA structured the subsidies, which are available to Marketplace enrollees with incomes from 100% to 400% of the federal poverty level, so that they could say that no one would have to pay a premium of more than 9.5% of their income (and many would pay less). The subsidies are calculated based on a benchmark premium in each geographic area: the second lowest-cost plan offered at the "silver" level of coverage. Enrollees are expected to pay a defined percentage of their income to enroll in that benchmark plan (ranging from 2% to 9.5% in 2014, with small changes over time based on increases in private insurance premiums relative to income), and a federal income tax credit covers the rest.

The result is that Marketplace enrollees eligible for subsidies—85% of all enrollees (KFF 2019c)—are insulated from premium increases. No matter how much the benchmark premium increases, federal premium subsidies rise to cover the difference, leaving enrollees paying approximately the same percentage of their income. (From a fiscal perspective, of course, federal spending for those subsidies increases.)

This subsidy structure has proven quite powerful. It has helped keep Marketplace enrollment stable, even in the face of large premium increases, protecting the market from a premium "death spiral" that would result if too many healthy people dropped out. It has also protected the Marketplace from the risk of so-called bare counties with no insurers participating at all. There is a strong incentive for an insurer to enter a market with no other plans, knowing that even with very high premiums, subsidized enrollees will not have to pay them.

The Repeal-and-Replace Debate

With the election of Donald Trump in 2016 and Republicans in charge of both the House and the Senate, "repeal and replace" of the ACA became a top priority going into 2017. It was during this period that the ACA exhibited its political resilience.

The House, after first abandoning the effort and then returning to it later, passed a version of repeal and replace that quickly proved quite controversial. The Congressional Budget Office (CBO) projected that the bill, which repealed the ACA's Medicaid expansion and substantially altered the premium subsidies, would result in 23 million more people uninsured by 2026 (CBO 2017a). Key to the bill's passage was a compromise worked out between moderate and conservative Republicans that would have allowed states to waive the ACA's benefit requirements and under certain circumstances community rating (which prohibits insurers from charging sicker people more than those who are healthy). President Trump, who celebrated the House bill's passage in a Rose Garden event, later called the bill "mean" (Kenny 2017). The Senate was ultimately unable to pass a bill and the repeal and replace effort died.

Many factors no doubt contributed to the failure of Republicans in Congress and President Trump to repeal and replace the ACA, but two elements of the law emerged as crucial to its staying power and decisive to moderate Republican swing votes in the Senate: the expansion of Medicaid and protections for people with preexisting conditions. Health industry groups and governors (including Republican governors) rallied to support the Medicaid expansion and oppose provisions that would have capped federal funding for the Medicaid program more generally and reduced spending substantially over time. People with preexisting conditions and their family members showed up at town hall meetings. Forty-five percent of nonelderly families have at least one adult with a preexisting condition that would have led to a decline of individual health insurance before the ACA (Claxton et al. 2019), and they proved to be a powerful and sympathetic voice in the debate.

Indeed, it was during the repeal-and-replace debate that the political tide for the ACA began to turn, with more Americans viewing it favorably than unfavorably (KFF 2019a). Republican efforts to repeal and replace the ACA, and in particular weaken protections for people with preexisting conditions, played a big role in the 2018 midterm election, helping Democrats retake the majority in the House.

Individual Mandate Repeal

While Republicans were unsuccessful at repealing the ACA itself, they did at the end of 2017 repeal the most unpopular part of the law, the so-called individual mandate. (Technically, the mandate to have health insurance or pay a penalty still exists, but the penalty is now zero.)

The ACA guaranteed access to coverage for people with preexisting conditions but needed to ensure that healthy people would enroll as well to avoid a premium death spiral. The law included a "carrot" (premium subsidies) as well as a "stick" (the individual mandate). CBO (2017b) predicted that repeal of the individual mandate penalty would push individual market premiums up by 10% and result in a significant increase in the number of people uninsured (4 million in 2019, rising to 13 million by 2027). (CBO later indicated that it believed the individual mandate was not as important as originally expected and repealing it would have more modest effects [Antos and Capretta 2018].)

Repeal of the individual mandate penalty did, in fact, have an upward effect on individual insurance market premiums (Kamal et al. 2018), but at least so far the effects on the number of people uninsured have not been as dire as expected. It may be that the ACA's "carrot" was more powerful than its "stick." Interestingly, repeal of the individual mandate may give the ACA even greater political resilience, jettisoning its most unpopular and controversial provision, as long as the Marketplace continues to function in a sustainable way.

Administrative Actions to Undermine the ACA

President Trump has taken a number of administrative actions to undermine the ACA, including expanding short-term plans that do not have to follow any of the ACA's rules and as a result offer much lower premiums to people without preexisting conditions (Levitt et al. 2018), as well as dramatically reducing outreach and funding for enrollment navigators (Pollitz, Tolbert, and Diaz 2019). A number of states have blunted these efforts by restricting short-term plans and maintaining funding for outreach in the exchanges they operate themselves (and additional states are moving to run their own exchanges).

Perhaps the president's highest-profile effort to undermine the health law was terminating federal payments to health insurers for cost-sharing reduction (CSR) subsidies. In addition to means-tested premium subsidies, the ACA required Marketplace insurers to offer reduced patient cost sharing for lower-income enrollees in silver-level plans. The federal government reimbursed insurers for the cost of providing this reduced cost sharing. The Republican majority in the House had sued the Obama administration, arguing that payments for the CSR subsidies were not properly authorized. President Trump threatened to cut off the CSR payments to insurers, saying it would cause the ACA to "implode" (Pear and Kaplan 2017). After numerous such threats, the president ultimately terminated the payments in October 2017.

However, rather than causing the ACA Marketplace to collapse, the cutoff of the cost-sharing subsidy payments allowed insurers to hold enrollees harmless, and even in some cases make them better off, through what became known as "silver loading." Insurers compensated for the loss of the federal cost-sharing subsidy payments by increasing silver premiums, based on the fact that the reduced cost sharing for lower-income enrollees is available only in silver plans. The premium for the lowest-cost silver plan increased by an average of 32% nationwide in 2018, compared to a 17% increase for less generous bronze plans and 18% for more generous gold plans (Semanskee, Claxton, and Levitt 2018).

Because the ACA's premium subsidies are tied to silver plans, those subsidies increased dramatically. Subsidized enrollees covered by silver plans were held harmless, and those choosing to sign up for bronze or gold plans saw their premiums net of subsidies fall. This effort to undermine the ACA backfired because of the structure of the law's premium subsidies. Enrollment among subsidized individuals has held steady at over 8 million people (Fehr, Cox, and Levitt 2019). Insurers are also returning to the ACA Marketplace and in many cases lowering premiums (Fehr, Kamal, and Cox 2019a), having increased profits substantially with recent premium increases (Fehr, Kamal, and Cox 2019b). Nationally, the benchmark premium decreased by an average of 3.5% in 2020.

Continuing Challenges

While the ACA has withstood multiple blows and remained standing, it is not working as well as its framers originally hoped and faces continuing challenges. With 14 states still not expanding Medicaid, 2.5 million uninsured people with incomes below poverty are not eligible for Medicaid but also not eligible for ACA premium subsidies (Garfield, Orgera, and Damico 2019). And, while people eligible for subsidies have been shielded from premium increases—some a result of the structure of the ACA, and others a result of actions taken by Congress and the Trump administration—middle-class people not eligible for subsidies have taken the full brunt of those increases. Individual market enrollment among those not receiving subsidies fell precipitously from 6.4 million in 2015 to 3.9 million in 2018 (Fehr, Cox, and Levitt 2019).

President Trump has continued to vow to repeal and replace the ACA after the 2020 election if he is reelected and Republicans control Congress (Cunningham 2019). And an ongoing lawsuit, supported by the Trump administration, threatens to overturn the ACA in its entirety, including protections for people with preexisting conditions and the expansion of Medicaid. However, with the knocks the law has taken and the resilience it has shown, the smart money would have to be on its continued existence.

■ ■ ■

Larry Levitt is executive vice president for health policy at the Kaiser Family Foundation. He has served as a senior health policy adviser to the White House, where he worked on the development of President Clinton's Health Security Act. He also has been the special assistant for health policy with California Insurance and a medical economist with Kaiser Permanente and has served in a number of positions in Massachusetts state government.
larryl@kff.org

References

Antos, Joseph R., and James C. Capretta. 2018. "CBO's Revised View of Individual Mandate Reflected in Latest Forecast." *Health Affairs Blog*, June 7. doi.org/10.1377/hblog20180605.966625.

CBO (Congressional Budget Office). 2017a. "H.R. 1628, American Health Care Act of 2017." May 24. www.cbo.gov/publication/52752.

CBO (Congressional Budget Office). 2017b. "Repealing the Individual Health Insurance Mandate: An Updated Estimate." November 8. www.cbo.gov/publication/53300.

Claxton, Gary, Cynthia Cox, Anthony Damico, Larry Levitt, and Karen Pollitz. 2019. "Pre-existing Condition Prevalence for Individuals and Families." Kaiser Family Foundation, October 7. www.kff.org/health-reform/issue-brief/pre-existing-condition-prevalence-for-individuals-and-families/.

Cunningham, Paige W. 2019. "The Health 202: Trump Now Says ACA Will Be Repealed and Replaced after 2020 Election." *Washington Post*, April 2. www.washingtonpost.com/news/powerpost/paloma/the-health202/2019/04/02/the-health-202-trump-now-says-aca-will-be-repealed-andreplaced-after-2020-election/5ca238811b326b0f7f38f2d7/.

Fehr, Rachel, and Cynthia Cox. 2020. "Individual Insurance Market Performance in Late 2019." Kaiser Family Foundation, January 6. www.kff.org/private-insurance/issue-brief/individual-insurance-market-performance-in-late-2019/.

Fehr, Rachel, Cynthia Cox, and Larry Levitt. 2019. "Data Note: Changes in Enrollment in the Individual Health Insurance Market through Early 2019." Kaiser Family Foundation, August 21. www.kff.org/private-insurance/issue-brief/data-note-changes-inenrollment-in-the-individual-health-insurance-market-through-early2019/.

Fehr, Rachel, Rabah Kamal, and Cynthia Cox. 2019a. "Insurer Participation on ACA Marketplaces, 2014–2020." Kaiser Family Foundation, November 21. www.kff.org/private-insurance/issue-brief/insurerparticipation-on-aca-marketplaces-2014-2020/.

Fehr, Rachel, Rabah Kamal, and Cynthia Cox. 2019b. "How ACA Marketplace Premiums Are Changing by County in 2020." Kaiser Family Foundation, November 7. www.kff.org/health-costs/issue-brief/how-aca-marketplace-premiums-are-changing-by-county-in-2020/.

Garfield, Rachel, Kendal Orgera, and Anthony Damico. 2019. "The Coverage Gap: Uninsured Poor Adults in States That Do Not Expand Medicaid." Kaiser Family Foundation, October 2. www.kff.org/medicaid/issue-brief/the-coverage-gap-uninsured-poor-adults-in-states-that-do-not-expand-medicaid/.

Goldstein, Amy. 2016. "Obamacare's Future in Critical Condition after Trump's Victory." *Washington Post*, November 9. www.washingtonpost.com/national/health-science/acas-future-incritical-condition-with-trumps-victory/2016/11/09/7c5587e8-a684-11e6ba59-a7d93165c6d4_story.html.

Kamal, Rabah, Cynthia Cox, Rachel Fehr, Marco Ramirez, Katherine Horstman, and Larry Levitt. 2018. "How Repeal of the Individual Mandate and Expansion of

Loosely Regulated Plans Are Affecting 2019 Premiums." Kaiser Family Foundation, October 30. www.kff.org/health-costs/issue-brief/how-repeal-of-the-individualmandate -and-expansion-of-loosely-regulated-plans-are-affecting-2019premiums/.

Kenny, Caroline. 2017. "Trump Confirms He Called Health Care Bill 'Mean' Victory." CNN, June 26. www.cnn.com/2017/06/25/politics/donaldtrump-confirms-mean -health-care/index.html.

KFF (Kaiser Family Foundation). 2019a. "Status of State Medicaid Expansion Deci- sions: Interactive Map." November 15. www.kff.org/medicaid/issue-brief/status-of -statemedicaid-expansion-decisions-interactive-map/.

KFF (Kaiser Family Foundation). 2019b. "Marketplace Average Benchmark Pre- miums." October 31. www.kff.org/health-reform/state-indicator/marketplace-average benchmarkpremiums/?currentTimeframe=0&sortModel=%7B%22colId22:%22 Location%22,%22sort%22:%22asc%22%7D.

KFF (Kaiser Family Foundation). 2019c. "Marketplace Plan Selections with Financial Assistance." March 27. www.kff.org/health-reform/state-indicator/marketplace -planselections-by-financial-assistance-status2/?currentTimeframe=0&sortModel=% 7B%22colId%22:%22Location%2,%22sort%22:%22asc%22%7D.

KFF (Kaiser Family Foundation). 2019d. "Status of State Medicaid Expansion Decisions: Interactive Map." November 15. www.kff.org/medicaid/issue-brief/status -of-statemedicaid-expansion-decisions-interactive-map/.

Levitt, Larry, Cynthia Cox, and Gary Claxton. 2016. "How ACA Marketplace Pre- miums Measure Up to Expectations." Kaiser Family Foundation, August 1. www .kff.org/healthreform/perspective/howaca-marketplace-premiums-measure-up-to -expectations/.

Levitt, Larry, Cynthia Cox, and Gary Claxton. 2017. "Insurer Financial Performance in the Early Years of the Affordable Care Act." Kaiser Family Foundation, April 21. www.kff.org/healthreform/issue-brief/insurer-financial-performance-in-the-early -years-of-theaffordable-care-act/.

Levitt, Larry, Rachel Fehr, Gary Claxton, Cynthia Cox, and Karen Pollitz. 2018. "Why Do Short-Term Health Insurance Plans Have Lower Premiums than Plans That Comply with the ACA?" Kaiser Family Foundation, November 1. www.kff.org /health-reform/issuebrief/why-do-short-term-health-insurance-plans-have-lower -premiumsthan-plans-that-comply-with-the-aca/.

Pear, Robert, and Thomas Kaplan. 2017. "Trump Threat to Obamacare Would Send Premiums and Deficits Higher." *New York Times*, August 15. www.nytimes.com /2017/08/15/us/politics/cbo-obamacare-costsharing-reduction-trump.html.

Pollitz, Karen, Jennifer Tolbert, and Maria Diaz. 2019. "Data Note: Limited Navigator Funding for Federal Marketplace States." Kaiser Family Foundation, November 13. www.kff.org/privateinsurance/issue-brief/data-note-further-reductions-in-navigator -fundingfor-federal-marketplace-states/.

Semanskee, Ashley, Gary Claxton, and Larry Levitt. 2018. "How Premiums Are Changing in 2018." Kaiser Family Foundation, November 20. www.kff.org/health -costs/issue-brief/how-premiums-arechanging-in-2018/.

US Supreme Court. 2012. *Syllabus: National Federation of Independent Business et al. v Sebelius, Secretary of Health and Human Services et al.* www.supremecourt .gov/opinions/11pdf/11-393c3a2.pdf.

Medicaid's Post-ACA Paradoxes

Colleen M. Grogan
University of Chicago

Abstract Medicaid's experience one decade after the passage of the Affordable Care Act represents extreme divergence across the American states in health care access and utilization, policy designs that either expand or restrict eligibility, and delivery model reforms. The past decade has also witnessed a growing ideological divide about the very purpose and intent of the Medicaid program and its place within the US health care system. While liberal-leaning states have actively embraced the program and used it to expand health coverage to working adults and families as an effort to improve health and prevent poverty and the insecurity and instability that comes with high medical costs (evictions, bankruptcy), conservative states have actively rejected this expanded idea of Medicaid and argued instead that the program should revert back to its "original" purpose and be used only for the "truly" needy. This article highlights several paradoxes within Medicaid that have led to this growing bifurcation, and it concludes by shedding light on important targets for future reform.

Keywords Medicaid, ACA, politics

> It was the best of times, it was the worst of times, it was the age of
> wisdom, it was the age of foolishness, it was the epoch of belief, it was
> the epoch of incredulity, it was the season of light, it was the season of
> darkness, it was the spring of hope, it was the winter of despair.
> —Charles Dickens, *A Tale of Two Cities*

Dickens's quote may suffer from overuse, but it is nonetheless a very accurate description of Medicaid's experience one decade after the passage of the Affordable Care Act (ACA). The past 10 years has witnessed the most dramatic expansion in the Medicaid program since it was enacted in 1965: 25.5 million Americans were enrolled in the program over this time

Journal of Health Politics, Policy and Law, Vol. 45, No. 4, August 2020
DOI 10.1215/03616878-8255541 © 2020 by Duke University Press

period, and today the program as a whole covers 21% of Americans (65.2 million in 2017), up from 13% (39.5 million) in 2008 (Kaiser Family Foundation 2019b).

At the same time, the past decade has witnessed a growing partisan divide about the very purpose and intent of the Medicaid program and its place within the US health care system. While Democratic-controlled states have actively embraced the program and used it to expand health coverage to working adults and families as an effort to improve health and to prevent poverty and the insecurity and instability that comes with high medical costs (evictions, bankruptcy), Republican-controlled states have actively rejected this expanded idea of Medicaid and argued instead that the program should revert back to its "original" purpose and be used only for the "truly" needy.

Of course, there are nuances amid the extremes. Some Republican-controlled states have enacted the Medicaid expansion, and Democratic-controlled states are just as likely as Republican-controlled states to embrace contracting with private managed care plans. In this article, I highlight several paradoxes within Medicaid that have led to a growing ideological bifurcation, to shed light on important targets for future reform.

Medicaid and Health Equity

The Best of Times

The ACA allowed states to expand Medicaid eligibility to nonelderly adults with incomes up to 138% of the federal poverty level (about $16,650 for individuals or $33,950 for a family of four in 2017). As of November 2019, 37 states have expanded Medicaid (including the District of Columbia and 3 states—Idaho, Utah, and Nebraska—that have adopted through referendum but have not yet implemented expansion), while 14 states have not (Kaiser Family Foundation 2019e). For states that expanded Medicaid, the overwhelming evidence suggests that expansion is linked to gains in coverage and improvements in access, financial security, and selected health outcomes.[1] Although there were (and remain) concerns about whether Medicaid would have sufficient capacity to serve the increased number of enrollees, and the findings on provider capacity are mixed, the majority of studies confirm that access to care and utilization of services has increased substantially in expansion states (Antonisse et al.

---

1. Two systematic reviews summarize the evidence to date: Antonisse et al. 2019 and Mazurenko et al. 2018.

2019; Mazurenko et al. 2018). Even very vulnerable "hard-to-reach" populations have gained access to coverage in Medicaid expansion states, including people with substance use disorders, people with HIV, and low-income adults diagnosed with depression or cancer (Antonisse et al. 2019).

The Medicaid expansion has also been able to fulfill a fundamental goal of insurance coverage: to protect individuals from financial liability when care is needed. Several studies demonstrate that financial security has improved among Medicaid enrollees in expansion states, and as a result, positive spillover effects are also realized: reductions in the poverty rate, personal bankruptcy, and evictions (Allen et al. 2019; Antonisse et al. 2019; Zewde and Wimer 2019). Fewer studies have been able to assess health outcomes, but self-reported health status has also improved (Allen et al. 2019; Antonisse et al. 2019; Zewde and Wimer 2019).

The Worst of Times

Given these findings of improved access to care and financial well-being for poor and low-income individuals, it is all the more appalling that millions of Americans remain uninsured in states that have refused to expand the Medicaid program. This gap in coverage left over 3 million Americans uninsured when the Medicaid expansion would have been fully enacted in 2014, and still nearly 2.5 million in 2017 (Garfield and Damico 2015).[2] This lack of coverage means different things to different people, but if you are sick and uninsured it almost certainly means that you do not have adequate access to the care you need. Especially in the midst of the opioid epidemic, for example, this means that people in nonexpansion states are less likely to get life-saving treatments (Grogan et al. 2020).

Medicaid Policy Innovations

The Age of Wisdom

Although researchers have long identified social factors such as income, education, and housing as crucially affecting health outcomes (Gottlieb, Wing, and Adler 2017), only in the last decade, with the onset of the Medicaid expansion, have states begun to invest in social needs. States

2. These figures represent only the so-called Medicaid gap—those not covered because states have not adopted the ACA Medicaid expansion. There are many more uninsured: nearly 28 million in 2017 (see Kaiser Family Foundation 2019b).

realize that Medicaid is uniquely positioned to support social needs, given its central role in providing coverage to low-income Americans (Alderwick, Hood-Ronick, and Gottlieb 2019). Under current Medicaid policy, states have the option to provide basic social supports to Medicaid enrollees, such as food or housing resources. Many states—Republican and Democrat alike—are using their contracts with managed care organizations (MCOs) to encourage or require referrals to address patients' social needs. In particular, in 2018, 16 states required MCOs to screen enrollees for social needs, and an additional 10 states encouraged the screening. Moreover, a survey of Medicaid MCOs revealed that over three-fourths of plans were undertaking activities to address housing needs, 73% were addressing nutrition, 51% education, and 31% employment needs (Hinton et al. 2019).

States can also apply for 1115 waivers to use Medicaid funds to invest in more intensive social interventions that often utilize health and social service partnerships. Several states have received such waivers to address patients' social needs (Kaiser Family Foundation 2019a). Early evidence of these initiatives in Oregon and Colorado suggests improvements in quality, controlling costs and reducing health disparities (McConnell et al. 2017; Muoto et al. 2016).

The Age of Foolishness

At the same time that more states are investing in addressing social needs, several Republican-led states are implementing policy reforms that focus on individual behaviors of particular Medicaid recipients, with the intent to increase personal responsibility, rooted in questions about whether certain low-income Americans deserve public coverage (Grogan, Singer, and Jones 2017; Vulimiri et al. 2019). As of November 2019, 7 states had approved work requirements, which require work as a condition of eligibility for Medicaid; 10 states required premium payments, including receipt of payment before coverage begins or a lock-out period (e.g., 6 months in Indiana) if premiums are not paid; and 7 states have received waivers to increase copays above previously allowed levels, and/or healthy behavior incentives tied to premiums or cost sharing (Kaiser Family Foundation 2019a).

Early data suggest these policy designs result in many individuals losing their Medicaid coverage. After Arkansas implemented its work requirement, 18,000 people were disenrolled from the program (Rudowitz,

Musumeci, and Hall 2019). Other studies found cost-related barriers due to Indiana's lock-out period if required payments were not deposited in health savings accounts. Although coverage has expanded in the state, its coverage gains are significantly less than in traditional expansion states because of these restrictions (Freedman, Richardson, and Simon 2018; Sommers et al. 2018). There are also serious concerns about how states will consider work requirements for people who are not officially classified as "disabled" but have behavioral health issues, such as opioid use disorder, or other chronic health conditions that make work requirements particularly challenging to fulfill (Wen, Saloner, and Cummings 2019).

Medicaid Political Polarization

The Epoch of Belief

When Medicaid was first enacted in 1965, political discourse and the actual eligibility rules, which tied Medicaid eligibility to cash assistance programs, described Medicaid as appropriate for certain categories of poor people—the elderly, blind and disabled, and poor (largely single-headed) families with dependent children. For those favoring national health insurance at the time, Medicaid was seen as a residual, stigmatizing program that could be dispensed when Medicare was extended to all Americans. However, among conservatives opposing national health insurance, Medicaid was viewed as appropriately restrictive because, if a person is poor but able-bodied, that person should be working and purchase private health insurance (or receive employer-sponsored health benefits) (Grogan and Patashnik 2003a, 2003b).

Of course, the assumption that working adults in low-wage jobs either received health benefits or earned enough to purchase health insurance was never true, but the rhetoric (and perhaps the actual belief) persisted in those early years. That all began to change in the 1980s with a set of incremental expansions that eventually extended coverage to all children under the federal poverty level (FPL) by 1990. The State Children's Health Insurance Program (SCHIP) was passed in 1997, which allowed states to expand Medicaid coverage to uninsured children of working parents up to 250% of the FPL. These efforts were largely bipartisan under a growing consensus that health insurance was necessary not only for those not working but also to prevent those working in lower-wage jobs from falling into poverty due to high medical expenses. SCHIP was viewed as particularly important for decoupling Medicaid from cash assistance and ushering in a growing ideological acceptance that low-income persons should have access to health insurance regardless of work or welfare status. I describe this as "growing" because, although SCHIP extended coverage for children above the poverty level in families with working adults, and there was widespread acceptance of the importance of covering children (though at different income levels), using Medicaid to extend coverage to low-income parents was very uneven across the states, and almost no states covered childless adults. Nonetheless, many states took advantage of the coverage options allowed under SCHIP in the early 2000s period, and it suggested a willingness among states to consider a broader vision for Medicaid. Indeed, the passage of the ACA in 2010 could be viewed as part of this trajectory, since the ACA Medicaid expansion finally moved the program away from categorical distinctions and declared that all persons earning less than 138% FPL eligible for Medicaid (Grogan 2013; Thompson 2012).

The Epoch of Incredulity

While the ACA Medicaid expansion allowed Democratic-controlled states to embrace this broader ideological vision of Medicaid as a program to prevent poverty and promote health equity for low- and even middle-income Americans, it also ushered in a strong rejection of this vision. The *National Federation of Independent Business v. Sebelius* lawsuit supported by 25 states argued against the constitutionality of the ACA mandate to expand Medicaid (Kaiser Family Foundation 2019d), and the Supreme Court ruled in favor of the plaintiff. This was arguably the most significant event after passage of the ACA, not only because it left millions of Americans uninsured but also because it opened the possibility for conservative states to bargain with the federal government over how to extend coverage. Even when Republican-controlled (or dominated) states adopted the Medicaid expansion, they often did so under a rejection of the Medicaid program (Grogan, Singer, and Jones 2017). This has had very important political implications.

First, although the program is expanded—in terms of both coverage and public expenditures—conservatives have attempted to revert the program, in actual policy design and, politically, in the broader public mind's eye, back to a residual welfare program. The work requirement not only kicks those deemed able-bodied but not working off Medicaid but also pits one group of Medicaid recipients against another under classic tropes of welfare deservingness: The program is for the *truly needy*, not those who take advantage and don't want to work (Grogan, Singer, and Jones 2017). This is important because the success of retrenchment politics depends on whether a large constituency would fight against such actions, thus threatening the reelection prospects of officials in support of retrenchment (Pierson 1994). It was arguably not lost on conservatives, especially in poor southern states where Medicaid expansion would result in nearly a third of the state's population relying on the Medicaid program (Grogan 2013), that passage of the Medicaid expansion could create an entitlement politics for Medicaid with favorable political feedback effects: once the program expands, it is difficult to rescind expanded coverage (Grogan and Park 2017a, 2018). Thus, conservative states rejected an expanded public vision of Medicaid, even when they used public funds to expand, in favor of a highly fragmented, unequal program, which is presented as public insurance for the undeserving and private insurance for the deserving (Grogan and Park 2017a, 2018).

Second, as Mettler (2018) describes, there is already a serious disconnect between Americans' actual dependence on government and their perception of it. Because a great deal of the American welfare state is structured through the tax system, such as employer-sponsored health insurance, most Americans who depend on tax-subsidized benefits do not see the role of government in the provision of these benefits and do not perceive themselves as benefiting from government policies. In a similar process, after the passage of SCHIP almost all of the states changed the name of their Medicaid program (at least for the uninsured children's program) in an attempt to destigmatize the program, and the vast majority of states contract out with Medicaid MCOs, which tends to obscure the role of the state and presents Medicaid benefits as private insurance to enrollees. Yet, conservative policy designs and political framing take this process one step further by strategically treating different groups differently to bifurcate coalition politics. Conservative state actors are engaged in a political classification process, which actively portrays their reform efforts as "not Medicaid" but, rather, a private initiative that demands "consumer-driven personal responsibility." Under this frame, the role of the state is intentionally hidden, and public funds received from the federal government are strategically obscured (Grogan, Singer, and Jones 2017; Mayrl and Quinn 2017).

Third, Medicaid's ideological cleavage mirrors the extreme political polarization reflected across our formal political institutions (e.g., in the US Congress, in the courts, and across state legislatures) and American public opinion (Hare and Poole 2014; Shor and McCarty 2011). While numerous historical accounts explicate how the development of the US health care system has been racially biased (Gamble 1995; Smith 2016; Wailoo 2001), there is evidence that as public opinion about health care reform has become more partisan since the passage of the ACA, it has also become more racially biased (Tesler 2012, 2013). Tesler (2012) documents that the racial gap in support for public insurance has significantly widened over time, with whites much less supportive than blacks or Latinos. Similarly, although several studies confirm that the composition of race in the state has long impacted the generosity of Medicaid benefits (if a state has a higher proportion of whites, means-tested eligibility levels tend to be higher), recent studies suggest that public opinion about the Medicaid expansion is also racialized (Grogan and Park 2017b; Lanford and Quadagno 2015), in two ways: large differences in support levels by race, and state adoption decisions positively related to white opinion and not responding to non-white support levels (Grogan and Park 2017b). This racialization is related to partisan visions of Medicaid. Rather than embrace a growing, unified vision of Medicaid that minimizes differences across class and race, the conservative vision highlights racial difference and invites conflict.

Medicaid Delivery Model Reforms

The Season of Light

Similar to state investments in social needs, Medicaid waivers allowed under the ACA have also ushered in major delivery model reforms attempting to coordinate care, improve quality, and lower costs. Every state in the nation is experimenting with some type of Medicaid delivery model reform, such as accountable care organizations, primary care medical homes, and health homes (Kaiser Family Foundation 2019c). While the attention to reforming the delivery system for Medicaid is unprecedented, there is little evidence to date on the outcomes of these reform efforts.

The Season of Darkness

A long-standing concern about the Medicaid program is that many providers refuse to participate in the program. Although the proportion of primary care physicians' patient panels made up of adult Medicaid patients increased in expansion states, from 10% to nearly 14% (Neprash et al. 2018), most Medicaid patients still utilize the health care safety net for their care. In 2015, 20% of primary care physicians saw 60% of Medicaid patients (Neprash et al. 2018). While Medicaid patients might prefer to see safety net providers, especially federally qualified health centers that offer wrap-around services, such as language translation and transportation, audit studies also confirm that relatively few private providers are available for new Medicaid patients (Polsky et al. 2018). In addition, so-called narrow networks—plans that employ 30% or fewer physicians in their market—are much more common among Medicaid MCOs than among employer-based MCOs or MCOs on the ACA Marketplaces (Ndumele et al. 2018; Polsky et al. 2018). Although the percentage of Medicaid MCOs with narrow networks has declined, from a high of 42% in 2011 to 27% in 2015, still one in four Medicaid MCOs offered to enrollees has a limited number of providers available and high turnover rates, raising concerns about continuity of care in addition to lack of choice (Ndumele et al. 2018). In sum, the hope of providing so-called mainstream medical care to Medicaid recipients has never been realized, and the ACA has not substantially changed that reality of a dual system of care.

There is also concern that, with little state oversight, for-profit commercial MCOs operating in the Medicaid program are earning significant profit margins (Herman 2016). The for-profit sector in Medicaid is substantial. Already by 2009, 41% of Medicaid MCO members were enrolled in publicly traded plans (McCue 2012). While the profit levels are concerning, there is almost no evidence to date about how Medicaid recipients fair in for-profit MCOs (especially post-ACA) relative to nonprofit plans.

The increase in public ACA funding has meant significant profits not only for many private organizations in the health care industry but also for private equity investors as well. Industries where Medicaid is the major funder of care (e.g., long-term care and home health care services, and behavioral health) have been a particularly lucrative target. For example, Medicaid is the largest payer for addiction treatment (Andrews et al. 2018), and private equity investments in behavioral health increased 24% in deal volume in just one year, amounting to $2.9 billion investments in treatment facilities in 2016 (Whalen and Cooper 2017). Private equity investment in the nursing home industry resulted in many facilities in large for-profit chains closing and laying off employees, while private equity executives and investors received substantial earnings (Appelbaum and Batt 2014; Baker 2019; Bos and Harrington 2017). Despite some murmurings of the need to regulate the private equity markets, especially as they have impacted needed medical facilities and services, the industry remains almost completely unregulated (Appelbaum and Batt 2014; Baker 2019; Bos and Harrington 2017).

Medicaid's Future

Spring of Hope to Winter of Despair

For those who had been fighting for universal coverage in the United States for a long time, the passage of the ACA in the spring of 2010 represented a time of hope. As many have written, we had not seen such a significant reform since the passage of Medicare and Medicaid in 1965 (Grogan, 2011a). These hopes were quickly dashed, however, with the immediate, virulent conservative backlash against the ACA and the Supreme Court ruling overturning the Medicaid mandate. After 6 full years of demonization of the ACA, we had clearly reached the winter of despair in 2017, when the ACA was saved only by the now famous thumbs-down vote of one notable senator, John McCain.

Back to Hope?

And yet, the ACA was saved in part because, for the first time since 2010, more Americans reported feeling favorable about the ACA than unfavorable, and although a partisan divide remained, by the summer of 2017 there was much less support for the repeal-and-replace bills even among Republicans (Kirzinger et al. 2017). Indeed, because Medicaid retrenchment was the centerpiece of the Republican ACA repeal efforts, one of the key arguments against it, even among members in their own party, was the impact repeal would have on their base. Because Medicaid has expanded over time, even in conservative states, and the Republican Party's core constituents include working-class voters, who ironically rely on the program for a vital source of financial protection and access to care, a sizable portion of the Republican base was against repeal and the significant cuts proposed to Medicaid. In summer of 2017, three-fourths of the general public (74%) held a favorable view of Medicaid, but 61% of Republicans also held a favorable view (Kaiser Family Foundation 2017).

Some have interpreted the mobilization against repeal as evidence that Medicaid has become entrenched and is on the path toward more political stability. This might be true, but others point out that we were just one vote short of repealing the ACA despite mobilization against it (Hacker and Pierson 2018; Patashnik and Oberlander 2018). It is clear that, as the Republican Party has moved further to the right ideologically, its members have been more willing to attack Medicaid—despite its popularity—as a welfare program (Rosenbaum 2018).[3] And, the increase in inequality in terms of how states treat their Medicaid enrollees, the racialization of Medicaid, private profits in Medicaid, and strategic efforts to obscure or make visible the states' role in Medicaid may also make it more difficult to create broad coalitions across race and class to fight against future attempts to retrench.

Can anything be done in light of these recent post-ACA trends? Underlying conservative efforts to radically reform the Medicaid program are false dichotomous portrayals of reform: "Promote private insurance and reduce the role of government." The "non-Medicaid" waiver reforms produce only a rhetorical elimination of government. When Republican-led states obtain waivers to enact a supposedly "non-Medicaid" expansion, they draw down the same federal subsidies that Democrat-led states use to expand Medicaid. Democratic states are just as likely as Republican states to contract with Medicaid MCOs, and when their Medicaid enrollees sign up for private plans, public funds subsidize the coverage.

Under "private" frames, the role of the state is intentionally hidden and public funds received from the federal government are strategically obscured. While Medicaid is defined as "public" and conservatives use old welfare tropes to describe enrollees on Medicaid, the health care system that middle- and upper-income Americans are said to rely on is repeatedly described as "predominantly private"—despite an estimated $437 billion in tax-exempt subsidies for employer-based health insurance in 2019 (Grogan 2015). In reality, the US health care system reflects a complete interdependence between private and public sectors (Grogan 2011b). Even Pauly (2019), writing for the conservative American Enterprise Institute, calculated that nearly 80% of health care dollars are government directed in some way, which fuels the growth in private-sector delivery and administration. Thus, labeling a program as "public" or "private" is a political construction and should be understood as part of a political (often partisan) struggle. As such, it is politically important to reveal some basic truths: first, the extent to which all Americans—across the income distribution—rely on public subsidies to obtain health care coverage, and second, the extent to which the financial industry (and therefore the extremely wealthy) are profiting off of the American health care system, while many Americans continue to struggle to access care and pay their medical bills.

---

3. For an explanation of Republican strategy around Medicaid related to the opioid epidemic, see Grogan et al. 2020.

■ ■ ■

Colleen M. Grogan is a professor at the University of Chicago in the School of Social Service Administration. Her research interests include health policy, health politics, and the American welfare state. She has written extensively on the history and current politics of the US Medicaid program. She is completing a book manuscript titled *The Rise of America's Conservative Health Care State*, which examines the historical development of political strategies and motivations behind hiding the role of government in the US health care system. She is co-associate editor for the health policy section of the *American Journal of Public Health*.
cgrogan@uchicago.edu

References

Alderwick, Hugh, Carlyn M. Hood-Ronick, and Laura M. Gottlieb. 2019. "Medicaid Investments to Address Social Needs in Oregon and California." *Health Affairs* 38, no. 5: 774–81.

Allen, Heidi L., Erica Ellason, Naomi Zewde, and Tal Gross. 2019. "Can Medicaid Expansion Prevent Housing Evictions?" *Health Affairs* 38, no. 9: 1451–57.

Andrews, Christina M., Colleen M. Grogan, Bikki Tran Smith, Amanda J. Abraham, Harold A. Pollack, Keith Humphreys, Melissa A. Westlake, and Peter D. Friedman. 2018. "Medicaid Benefits for Addiction Treatment Expanded after Implementation of the Affordable Care Act." *Health Affairs* 37, no. 8: 1216–22.

Antonisse, Larisa, Rachel Garfield, Robin Rudowitz, and Madeline Guth. 2019. "The Effects of Medicaid Expansion under the ACA: Updated Findings from a Literature Review." Kaiser Family Foundation, August 15. www.kff.org/medicaid/issue-brief /the-effects-of-medicaid-expansion-under-the-aca-updated-findings-from-a-literature -review-august-2019/.

Appelbaum, Eileen, and Rosemary Batt. 2014. *Private Equity at Work: When Wall Street Manages Main Street*. New York: Russell Sage Foundation.

Baker, Jim. 2019. "Adverse Reaction: How Will the Flood of Private Equity Money into Health Care Providers Impact Access to, Cost, and Quality of Care?" Private Equity Stakeholder Project, November. pestakeholder.org/wp-content/uploads /2019/11/Adverse-Reaction-PE-Investment-in-Health-Care-PESP-110619.pdf.

Bos, Aline, and Charlene Harrington. 2017. "What Happens to a Nursing Home Chain When Private Equity Takes Over? A Longitudinal Case Study." *International Health Economics and Finance* 54: 1–10.

Freedman, Seth, Lilliard Richardson, and Kosali I. Simon. 2018. "Learning from Waiver States: Coverage Effects under Indiana's HIP Medicaid Expansion." *Health Affairs* 37, no. 6: 936–43.

Gamble, Vanessa Northington. 1995. *Making a Place for Ourselves: The Black Hospital Movement 1920–1945*. New York: Oxford University Press.

Garfield, Rachel, and Anthony Damico. 2015. "The Coverage Gap: Uninsured Poor Adults in States That Do Not Expand Medicaid—An Update." Kaiser Family Foundation, Issue Brief, October. nationaldisabilitynavigator.org/wp-content/uploads/news-items/KFF_coverage-gap-uninsured-in-states-not-expanding-medicaid.pdf.

Gottlieb, Laura M., Holly Wing, and Nancy E. Adler. 2017. "A Systematic Review of Interventions on Patients' Social and Economic Needs." *American Journal of Preventive Medicine* 53, no. 5: 719–29.

Grogan, Colleen M., ed. 2011a. "Introduction to Special Issue: Critical Essays on Health Care Reform." Special issue, *Journal of Health Politics, Policy and Law* 36, no. 3: 369–71.

Grogan, Colleen M., ed. 2011b. "You Call It Public, I Call It Private, Let's Call the Whole Thing Off?" Special issue, *Journal of Health Politics, Policy and Law* 36, no. 3: 401–11.

Grogan, Colleen M. 2013. "Medicaid: Designed to Grow" In *Health Politics and Policy*, 5th ed., edited by James Morone and Daniel Ehlke, 142–63. Stamford, CT: Cengage Learning.

Grogan, Colleen M. 2015. "The Role of the Private Sphere in US Healthcare Entitlements: Increased Spending, Weakened Public Mobilization, and Reduced Equity." *Forum* 13, no. 1: 119–42.

Grogan, Colleen M., Clifford S. Bersamira, Phillip M. Singer, Bikki Tran Smith, Harold A. Pollack, Christina M. Andrews, and Amanda J. Abraham. 2020. "Are Policy Strategies to Address the Opioid Epidemic Partisan? A View from the States." *Journal of Health Politics, Policy and Law* 45 no. 2: 277–309.

Grogan, Colleen M., and Eric Patashnik. 2003a. "Between Welfare Medicine and Mainstream Program: Medicaid at the Political Crossroads." *Journal of Health Politics, Policy and Law* 28, no. 5: 821–58.

Grogan, Colleen M., and Eric Patashnik. 2003b. "Universalism within Targeting: Nursing Home Care, the Middle Class, and the Politics of the Medicaid Program." *Social Service Review* 77, no. 1: 51–71.

Grogan, Colleen M., and Sunggeun Park. 2017a. "The Politics of Medicaid: Most Americans Are Connected to the Program, Support Its Expansion, and Do Not View It as Stigmatizing." *Milbank Quarterly* 95, no. 4: 749–82.

Grogan, Colleen M., and Sunggeun Park. 2017b. "The Racial Divide in State Medicaid Expansions." *Journal of Health Politics, Policy and Law* 42, no. 3: 539–72.

Grogan, Colleen M., and Sunggeun Park. 2018. "Medicaid Retrenchment Politics: Fragmented or Unified?" *Journal of Social Policy and Aging* 30, nos. 3–4: 372–99.

Grogan, Colleen M., Phillip M. Singer, and David K. Jones. 2017. "Rhetoric and Reform in Waiver States." *Journal of Health Politics, Policy and Law* 42, no. 2: 247–84.

Hacker, Jacob S., and Paul Pierson. 2018. "The Dog That Almost Barked: What the ACA Repeal Fight Says about the Resilience of the American Welfare State." *Journal of Health Politics, Policy and Law* 43, no. 4: 551–77.

Hare, Christopher, and Keith T. Poole. 2014. "The Polarization of Contemporary American Politics." *Polity* 46, no. 3: 411–29.

Herman, Bob. 2016. "Medicaid's Unmanaged Managed Care." *Modern Healthcare*, April 30. www.modernhealthcare.com/article/20160430/MAGAZINE/304309980 /medicaid-s-unmanaged-managed-care.

Hinton, Elizabeth, Robin Rudowitz, Maria Diaz, and Natalie Singer. 2019. "Ten Things to Know about Medicaid Managed Care." Kaiser Family Foundation, Issue Brief, December. files.kff.org/attachment/Issue-Brief-10-Things-to-Know-about -Medicaid-Managed-Care.

Kaiser Family Foundation. 2017. "Data Note: Ten Charts about Public Opinion on Medicaid." June. www.kff.org/medicaid/poll-finding/data-note-10-charts-about -public-opinion-on-medicaid/.

Kaiser Family Foundation. 2019a. "Approved Section 1115 Medicaid Waivers." www .kff.org/other/state-indicator/approved-section-1115-medicaid-waivers/?current Timeframe=0andsortModel=%7B%22colId%22:%22Location%22,%22sort%22:% 22asc%22%7D (accessed November 24, 2019).

Kaiser Family Foundation. 2019b. "Health Insurance Coverage of the Total Population." www.kff.org/other/state-indicator/total-population/?currentTime frame=0andsortModel=%7B%22colId%22:%22Location%22,%22sort%22:%22 asc%22%7D (accessed November 14, 2019).

Kaiser Family Foundation 2019c. "Mapping Medicaid Delivery System and Payment Reform." October 18. www.kff.org/interactive/delivery-system-and-payment-reform/.

Kaiser Family Foundation. 2019d. "States' Positions in the Affordable Care Act Case at the Supreme Court." State Health Facts. www.kff.org/health-reform/state-indicator /state-positions-on-aca-case/?currentTimeframe=0andsortModel=%7B%22colId% 22:%22Location%22,%22sort%22:%22asc%22%7D (accessed November 24, 2019).

Kaiser Family Foundation. 2019e. "Status of State Medicaid Expansion Decisions: Interactive Map." www.kff.org/medicaid/issue-brief/status-of-state-medicaid -expansion-decisions-interactive-map/ (accessed November 14, 2019).

Kirzinger, Ashley, Bianca DiJulio, Liz Hamel, Bryan Wu, and Mollyann Brodie. 2017. "Kaiser Health Tracking Poll—June 2017: ACA, Replacement Plan, and Medic- aid." Kaiser Family Foundation, June 23. www.kff.org/health-reform/poll-finding /kaiser-health-trackingpoll-june-2017-aca-replacement-plan-and-medicaid/.

Lanford, Daniel, and Jill Quadagno. 2015. "Implementing Obamacare: The Politics of Medicaid Expansion under the Affordable Care Act of 2010." *Sociological Per- spectives* 59, no. 3: 619–39.

Mayrl, Damon, and Sarah Quinn. 2017. "Beyond the Hidden American State: Clas- sification Struggles and the Politics of Recognition." In *The Many Hands of the State*, edited by Kimberly J. Morgan and Ann Shola Orloff, 58–80. New York: Cambridge University Press.

Mazurenko, Olena, Casey P. Balio, Rajender Agarwal, Aaron E. Carroll, and Nir Menachemi. 2018. "The Effects of Medicaid Expansion under the ACA: A Sys- tematic Review." *Health Affairs* 37, no. 6: 944–50.

McConnell, K. John, Stephanie Renfro, Benjamin K. Chan, Thomas H. A. Meath, Aaron Mendelson, Deborah J. Cohen, Jeanette A. Waxmonsky, Dennis McCarty, Neal Wallace, and Richard C. Lindrooth. 2017. "Early Performance in Medicaid

Accountable Care Organizations: A Comparison of Oregon and Colorado." *JAMA Internal Medicine* 177, no. 4: 538–45.

McCue, Mike. 2012. "Financial Performance of Health Plans in Medicaid Managed Care." *Medicare and Medicaid Research Review* 2, no. 2: E1–E10. www.cms.gov /mmrr/Downloads/MMRR2012_002_02_A07.pdf.

Mettler, Suzanne. 2018. *The Government–Citizen Disconnect.* New York: Russell Sage Foundation.

Muoto, Ifeoma, Jeff Luck, Jangho Yoon, Stephanie Bernell, and Jonathan Snowden. 2016. "Oregon's Coordinated Care Organizations Increased Timely Prenatal Care Initiation and Decreased Disparities." *Health Affairs* 35, no. 9: 1625–32.

Ndumele, Chima D., Becky Staiger, Joseph S. Ross, and Mark J. Schlesinger. 2018. "Network Optimization and the Continuity of Physicians in Medicaid Managed Care." *Health Affairs* 37, no. 6: 929–35.

Neprash, Hannah T., Anna Zink, Joshua Gray, and Katherine Hempstead. 2018. "Datawatch: Physicians' Participation in Medicaid Increased Only Slightly Following Expansion." *Health Affairs* 37, no. 7: 1087–91.

Patashnik, Eric M., and Jonathan Oberlander. 2018. "After Defeat: Conservative Postenactment Opposition to the ACA in Historical-Institutional Perspective." *Journal of Health Politics, Policy and Law* 43, no. 4: 651–82.

Pauly, Mark. 2019. "Will Health Care's Immediate Future Look a Lot Like the Recent Past? More Public-Sector Funding, But More Private-Sector Delivery and Administration." American Enterprise Institute, June. www.aei.org/research-products/report /health-care-public-sector-funding/.

Pierson, Paul. 1994. *Dismantling the Welfare State? Reagan, Thatcher, and the Politics of Retrenchment.* Cambridge: Cambridge University Press.

Polsky, Daniel, Molly K. Candon, Paula Chatterjee, and Xinwei Chen. 2018. "Datawatch: Scope of Primary Care Physicians' Participation in the Health Insurance Marketplaces." *Health Affairs* 37, no. 8: 1252–56.

Rosenbaum, Sara. 2018. "The (Almost) Great Unraveling." *Journal of Health Politics, Policy and Law* 43, no. 4: 579–603.

Rudowitz, Robin, MaryBeth Musumeci, and Cornelia Hall. 2019. "February State Data for Medicaid Work Requirements in Arkansas." Kaiser Family Foundation, March 25. www.kff.org/medicaid/issue-brief/state-data-for-medicaid-work-requirements -in-arkansas/.

Shor, Boris, and Nolan McCarty. 2011. "The Ideological Mapping of American Legislatures." *American Political Science Review* 105, no. 3: 530–51.

Smith, David John. 2016. *The Power to Heal: Civil Rights, Medicare, and the Struggle to Transform America's Health Care System.* Nashville, TN: Vanderbilt University Press.

Sommers, Benjamin D., Carrie E. Fry, Robert J. Blendon, and Arnold M. Epstein. 2018. "New Approaches in Medicaid: Work Requirements, Health Savings Accounts, and Health Care Access." *Health Affairs* 37, no. 7: 1099–1108.

Tesler, Michael. 2012. "The Spillover of Racialization into Health Care: How President Obama Polarized Public Opinion by Racial Attitudes and Race." *American Journal of Political Science* 56, no. 3: 690–704.

Tesler, Michael. 2013. "The Return of Old-Fashioned Racism to White Americans' Partisan Preferences in the Early Obama Era." *Journal of Politics* 75, no. 1: 110–23.

Thompson, Frank J. 2012. *Medicaid Politics: Federalism, Policy Durability, and Health Reform*. Washington, DC: Georgetown University Press.

Vulimiri, Madhulika, William K. Bleser, Robert S. Saunders, Farrah Madanay, Connor Moseley, F. Hunter McGuire, Peter A. Ubel, Aaron McKethan, Mark McClellan, and Charlene A. Wong. 2019. "Engaging Beneficiaries in Medicaid Programs That Incentivize Health-Promoting Behaviors." *Health Affairs* 38, no. 3: 431–39.

Wailoo, Keith. 2001. *Dying in the City of the Blues: Sickle Cell Anemia and the Politics of Race and Health*. Chapel Hill: University of North Carolina Press.

Wen, Hefei, Brendan Saloner, and Janet R. Cummings. 2019. "Behavioral and Other Chronic Conditions among Adult Medicaid Enrollees: Implications for Work Requirements." *Health Affairs* 38, no. 4: 660–67.

Whalen, Jeanne, and Laura Cooper. 2017. "Private-Equity Pours Cash into Opioid-Treatment Sector." *Wall Street Journal*, September 2. www.wsj.com/articles/opioid-crisis-opens-opportunities-for-private-equity-firsts-1504353601.

Zewde, Naomi, and Christopher Wimer. 2019. "Antipoverty Impact of Medicaid Growing with State Expansion over Time." *Health Affairs* 38, no. 1: 132–38.

States, Federalism, and Medicaid
The Administrative Presidency, Waivers, and the Affordable Care Act

Michael K. Gusmano
Frank J. Thompson
Rutgers University

Abstract Within the American system of shared power among institutions, the executive branch has played an increasingly prominent policy role relative to Congress. The vast administrative discretion wielded by the executive branch has elevated the power of the president. Republican and Democratic presidents alike have employed an arsenal of administrative tools to pursue their policy goals: high-level appointments, administrative rule making, executive orders, proclamations, memoranda, guidance documents, directives, dear colleague letters, signing statements, reorganizations, funding decisions, and more. Presidents Obama and Trump employed most of these tools in an effort to shape the implementation and outcomes of the Affordable Care Act (ACA) during its first decade. This article focuses on the Obama and Trump administrations' use of comprehensive waivers to shape ACA implementation. The Obama administration had mixed success using waivers to convince Republican states to expand Medicaid. Compared to Obama, the Trump administration has found it harder to accomplish its policy goals through waivers, but if the courts support the Trump administration's work requirement and 1332 waiver initiatives, it would enable the president to use waivers to achieve an ever broader set of goals, including program retrenchment.

Keywords ACA, Medicaid, waivers

Within the American system of shared power among institutions, the executive branch has played an increasingly prominent policy role relative to Congress. The vast administrative discretion wielded by the executive branch has elevated the power of the president. The rise of an aggressive, partisan, multifaceted administrative presidency fueled especially by

Journal of Health Politics, Policy and Law, Vol. 45, No. 4, August 2020
DOI 10.1215/03616878-8255553   © 2020 by Duke University Press

Ronald Reagan in the 1980s, has meant that significant policy shifts often occur without congressional approval. Republican and Democratic presidents alike have employed an arsenal of administrative tools to pursue their policy goals (Thompson, Wong, and Rabe forthcoming). These include high-level appointments, administrative rulemaking, executive orders, proclamations, memoranda, guidance documents, directives, dear colleague letters, signing statements, reorganizations, funding decisions, and more (Howell 2003; Lewis 2008; Nathan 1983). Presidents Obama and Trump employed most of these tools in an effort to shape the implementation and outcomes of the Affordable Care Act (ACA) during its first decade. Our focus is on a tool particularly important in the context of federalism: program waivers. This article opens by briefly reviewing the role of waivers in health policy generally and with respect to the ACA more specifically. The next two sections then assay how the Obama administration sought to use waivers as a catalyst for the Medicaid expansion, and how the Trump administration employed this tool in an effort to depress Medicaid enrollments. We then address the strategic posture of the two presidential administrations toward the ACA's section 1332 waivers, which aim to provide states with opportunities to pursue alternative approaches to health reform. A final section assesses the degree to which the waiver strategies of the Obama and Trump administrations facilitated achievement of their respective policy goals.

Program Waivers as a Policy Tool

Waivers are congressional delegations of authority to the federal executive branch to permit selective deviations from the law. The use of waivers in health care was infrequent before President Clinton. Since that time, states have submitted and had approved hundreds of waivers, many of which allowed them to transform their Medicaid programs. States have obtained more focused waivers under section 1915 of the Medicaid statute in order to increase the proportion of long-term services and supports offered in the home and community rather than in institutions.

We focus on waivers that are broader in scope, more likely to kindle partisan differences and to be seen by presidents and state policy makers as vehicles for major policy action. In this, regard, waivers anchored in section 1115 of the Social Security Act, approved by Congress in 1962, give the federal executive branch substantial authority to experiment with alternative state approaches to program delivery. These waivers are supposed to generate policy learning by requiring that demonstrations be formally evaluated. Between the 1990s and the adoption of the ACA in 2010, 1115 waivers permitted states to shift most Medicaid enrollees from fee for service to managed care, expand Medicaid coverage to new cohorts of low-income adults, and reshape their health care infrastructures. About 80% of states had demonstration waivers approved or pending during the ACA's initial decade, with about one-third of federal Medicaid expenditures supporting waiver-based activities (GAO 2019a). These waivers figured prominently in the administrative strategies toward the ACA of both Presidents Obama and Trump.

The ACA added another major waiver to the tool box of the administrative presidency. Section 1332 of the ACA authorizes the Department of Health and Human Services and the Department of the Treasury to waive the law's insurance exchange provisions so that states may provide alternative approaches to expanding high-quality coverage in the individual and small-group health insurance markets. It requires state waiver proposals to offer insurance as comprehensive and affordable as ACA plans, and not to decrease the number of people who have coverage. The waivers must be authorized by state legislation and approved by the governor; they must not increase the federal deficit. Supporters of the ACA saw the 1332 waivers as an opportunity to explore other approaches to universal coverage. Officials in Vermont, for instance, planned to use a 1332 waiver to promote single-payer reform (McDonough 2015). But a president seeking to undermine the ACA may also turn to innovation waivers as a tool.

Different uses of demonstration and innovation waivers were on display during the ACA's first decade. President Obama used 1115 waivers as a platform for negotiating the ACA's Medicaid expansion in states that would otherwise resist such action. In dealing with the 1332 waivers he sought to establish guardrails that would make it hard for states to water down the ACA's insurance standards. The Trump administration's actions with respect to the demonstration and innovation waivers sought to substantially undermine the ACA. In the case of the Medicaid expansion population, the Trump administration invited states to submit 1115 waivers imposing work requirements and other administrative burdens on enrollees that would cause many of them to lose coverage. As for 1332 waivers, the Trump administration encouraged states to submit proposals that might not meet the ACA's requirements to cover people with preexisting conditions, provide the law's 10 essential health benefits, or cap the out-of-pocket expenses of enrollees.

Obama: Demonstration Waivers as Catalysts for Medicaid Expansion

The ACA's goal of expanding health insurance coverage depended heavily on Medicaid. The law mandated that, with certain exceptions, all nonelderly, nondisabled people with incomes up to 138% of the poverty line would qualify for Medicaid. It called for the federal government to pay the tab for the newly eligible for 3 years starting in 2014. In 2017, this federal match would decline, leveling off at 90% in 2020. States that refused to comply with this mandate risked having funding for their existing Medicaid program reduced. But in *National Federation of Independent Business v. Sebelius*, the Supreme Court in 2012 ruled that the federal government could *not* eliminate funding for existing Medicaid programs if states refused to join the ACA's Medicaid expansion. This decision effectively converted the expansion from a federal mandate to a state option and presented the Obama administration with the challenge of persuading resistant states to expand the program.

The partisan divisions over the ACA meant that the administrative presidency, rather than the career bureaucracy, led the negotiations between the federal and state governments. Both administrations saw the implementation and success (or failure) of the ACA as closely linked to broader party goals, so the White House wanted more direct involvement than was the case for many Medicaid waivers. In doing so, Obama faced the problem that Republicans dominated most state governments: in 2013, Republicans controlled the governorship and both houses of the legislature in 24 states; 6 of the 12 states with divided governments had Republican governors. National party leaders and related partisan networks urged these policy makers to shun more pragmatic policy and administrative considerations in weighing their responses to the ACA and instead join national partisan efforts to derail the law's implementation.

In waiver negotiations with governors, the Obama administration stood firm on certain matters. Several Republican governors pushed the Centers for Medicare and Medicaid Services (CMS) to accept a partial expansion of Medicaid, such as covering those up to 100% of the poverty line rather than 138%. In December 2012, however, the Obama administration announced that it would not approve partial measures. The White House gambled that, in doing so, the ACA's generous federal match, as well as lobbying pressures from providers and others, would eventually encourage most if not all states to expand Medicaid. Indeed, the administration did not merely hope that these groups would pressure state governments to expand Medicaid; it encouraged their mobilization.

Meanwhile, the Obama administration used section 1115 waiver authority to facilitate expansion. This included granting waivers to supportive states to jump-start implementation of the law prior to 2014. In late 2010, for instance, CMS approved a Medicaid waiver for California called "Bridge to Reform," which provided federal matching funds to counties in the state that got a head start implementing the ACA's Medicaid provisions. The Obama administration also sought to use waiver renewal processes to incentivize Medicaid expansion. It strove to phase out waivers in states such as Florida that had diverted Medicaid monies into subsidies for hospitals rather than insurance for individuals. It saw no need to continue the hospital pools when these states could address problems of uncompensated care by expanding Medicaid.

But the primary Medicaid expansion strategy of the Obama administration centered on encouraging state Republican policy makers to submit new waiver proposals. The interest of conservative policy makers in market-oriented waivers gave the Obama administration an opening. The waivers pursued by these states sought to push Medicaid more fully toward a model that stressed private insurance, competition among providers, individual choice, consumer empowerment, and personal responsibility. The market-oriented model in varying degrees emphasizes two broad themes.

One theme is individual choice and personal responsibility. This variant stresses that Medicaid enrollees will behave more responsibly if they have some "skin in the game" when making health care decisions, such as by paying premiums, having copays for services, or managing health savings accounts. It seeks to discourage "inappropriate" care through greater cost sharing when enrollees use hospital emergency departments for nonurgent services. It also uses economic incentives to reward enrollees if they engage in certain desired health care behaviors (e.g., waiving premiums if they get an annual wellness exam) or other activities such as employment training or work. Under Obama, Indiana, Michigan, and Montana received waivers emphasizing individual choice and personal responsibility as a condition for expanding Medicaid.

A second theme of some market-oriented waivers is premium assistance. This approach involves the use of Medicaid monies to purchase coverage from private insurance companies on the ACA's exchanges. The Obama administration approved waivers in Arkansas, Iowa, New Hampshire, and Pennsylvania (where a newly elected Democratic governor terminated the waiver in 2015) that stressed this kind of assistance. In varying degrees, these waivers allow individuals in the Medicaid expansion cohort to seek coverage on the exchanges rather than sign up for the state's Medicaid program. The Obama administration faced the challenge that insuring people on the exchanges would likely cost more than enrolling them in Medicaid, which violates the federal requirement that demonstration waivers be budget neutral. Following in the tradition of earlier presidents, the Obama administration finessed this problem by accepting generous assumptions from the states about the cost savings their waivers would produce.

In using waivers as carrots for Medicaid expansion, the Obama administration did not grant all state requests. It resisted efforts by Republican governors in Arizona, Indiana, Kentucky, Ohio, and Pennsylvania to impose work requirements on Medicaid applicants. In other cases, the Obama administration rejected enrollee cost sharing that it considered excessive; it declined some state measures that would increase the administrative burdens of Medicaid enrollment processes. The use of waivers as well as other policy dynamics led to slow but steady progress in increasing the number of Medicaid-expansion states. By the time Obama left office, 31 states and the District of Columbia had expanded Medicaid.

Trump: Demonstration Waivers as Catalysts for Enrollment Erosion

Like Obama, the Trump administration viewed 1115 waivers as a tool to pursue its policy goals without congressional action. This became particularly important after the Republican-controlled Congress failed to adopt a "repeal-and-replace" law in 2017. Even before that, in March Tom Price, secretary of health and human services at the time, sent a letter to all governors encouraging new 1115 waiver submissions (Price and Verma 2017). The letter endorsed premiums and other enrollee cost sharing, as well as fees penalizing enrollees who use hospital emergency departments for nonurgent care. It opened the door to state initiatives that would reverse Obama administration efforts to increase Medicaid take-up rates. For instance, it welcomed state restrictions on "presumptive eligibility," which health care providers had used to obtain Medicaid funding for uninsured patients who appeared to qualify for Medicaid but had not yet formally applied. The Trump administration's waiver themes emphasized work mandates, greater premiums, more extensive reporting, and a gaggle of other requirements for the able-bodied, nonelderly adults targeted by the ACA's Medicaid expansion. These requirements would greatly increase the administrative burdens on Medicaid applicants and beneficiaries and generally depress program enrollments (Moynihan, Herd, and Harvey 2015).

In November, Seema Verma, who had been confirmed as administrator of CMS, more fully developed these themes. Speaking at a meeting of state Medicaid directors, Verma (2017) promised a "new day" for Medicaid, stressing that the ACA had caused the program to stray from its core mission of helping society's most vulnerable members. Doing so had stretched "the safety net for some of our most fragile populations, many of whom are on waiting lists for critical home-care services while states enroll millions of newly eligible, able-bodied adults" at an enhanced match rate of 90%. Having portrayed the expansion population as undeserving and a threat to more meritorious cohorts of Medicaid enrollees, Verma went on to endorse state flexibility to impose work requirements on able-bodied adults. In her view, these requirements would help these enrollees "break the chains of poverty" and surmount "the soft bigotry of low expectations consistently espoused by the prior administration." Amplifying this theme, CMS prepared a new website that no longer included "increase and strengthen overall coverage of low-income individuals" as a Medicaid waiver goal (Cohen 2017). On January 11, 2018, CMS sent a letter to state Medicaid directors justifying work requirements on grounds that they would "promote better mental, physical and emotional health" for beneficiaries (CMS 2018).

As of December 2019, 10 states (Arizona, Arkansas, Indiana, Kentucky, Michigan, New Hampshire, Ohio, South Carolina, Utah, and Wisconsin) had obtained CMS approval for work requirement waivers, with another 8 awaiting the agency's decision on their proposals. (After the 2019 elections, Democratic governors in Kentucky and Virginia announced their intention to withdraw their respective work waivers.) All but 2 of the 18 states with approved or pending waivers had a Republican governor at the time of waiver submission; all but two had voted for Trump in the 2016 presidential election. Waiver proposals varied, but they typically mandated that a specified cohort of nonelderly, able-bodied adults be employed for at least 20 hours per week. The work requirements primarily targeted those gaining eligibility under the ACA's Medicaid expansion. But such non-expansion states as South Carolina and Wisconsin also won approval to impose them. "Work" generally encompassed such activities as employment, education or training, and job search. The waivers also tended to allow enrollees to meet the requirement through various forms of community engagement, such as volunteering with a nonprofit group.

While state work requirements would sap Medicaid enrollments, the degree of decline also depended on other administrative burdens embedded in the waivers. Reporting requirements comprised one such burden. These requirements become more burdensome if they must be done more frequently, call for more submitted information, or limit communication channels for enrollee reporting. Several of the approved work waivers featured burdensome reporting requirements. Arkansas, for instance, required able-bodied enrollees aged 19–49 to report the status of their work efforts on a monthly basis and limited the venues for communicating this information. Though many enrollees had no or limited computer skills, they had to report electronically through a special state web portal. If enrollees did not have access to the internet at home or through mobile devices, county offices would have portals available during work hours. To use the portal, an enrollee needed an e-mail address, a password unique to the portal, and a reference number that Medicaid officials had sent in a multipage letter. Once linked to the portal, enrollees had to click through several different screens to report their work and community engagement activities.

The requirement for electronic filing promised to pare the administrative costs of the work initiative. Although CMS does not take administrative costs into account in determining whether a waiver proposal is budget neutral, these costs tend to be substantial. Arkansas had incentive to rely exclusively on an electronic portal because the federal government covers 90% of state administrative costs for pertinent information system development while subsidizing only half of most other administrative costs (GAO 2019b).

This reporting structure precipitated declines in Medicaid enrollments. The Arkansas waiver stipulated that beneficiaries who failed to comply with work requirements for 3 months would be locked out of coverage for the remainder of the calendar year. In September, 3 months after waiver implementation began, state officials announced that over 4,300 people would lose coverage for failing to report. By the end of 2018, nearly 17,000 had lost coverage (Rudowitz, Musumeci, and Hall 2018).

Lock-out periods in many of the approved waivers also place burdens on enrollees. These periods refer to the length of time a beneficiary loses coverage for failure to comply with Medicaid requirements. For example, the Kentucky waiver established a 6–month disenrollment for beneficiaries who did not promptly report changes in income or employment status. Former enrollees could shorten the lock-out period by completing a financial or health literacy course.

Some of the approved waivers also impose new financial burdens on enrollees through cost-sharing provisions. Medicaid law permits some enrollee cost sharing but generally prohibits states from charging premiums to beneficiaries with incomes below 150% of the poverty line. Some of the approved waivers departed from that norm. For instance, Kentucky's waiver required enrollees who were at 0–25% of the poverty line to pay a monthly premium of $1; those in the 25–50% range had to pay $4 monthly.

CMS was not responsive to all initiatives embedded in the state waiver proposals. It did not, for instance, sign off on Wisconsin's proposal to impose mandatory drug screening for poor, childless, able-bodied Medicaid applicants ages 19–64, nor did it accept that state's proposal to establish a 4–year time limit on eligibility for this Medicaid cohort. CMS also turned down several state proposals to reduce Medicaid eligibility for the expansion population from 138% of the poverty line to 100%. While showing some restraint with these and other requests, however, the Trump administration's waiver approvals clearly threatened to erode Medicaid enrollments, and litigation to block these initiatives soon emerged.

Opponents filed suits over 2 years to derail the work requirement waivers, initially in Kentucky and Arkansas and then in New Hampshire, Indiana, and Michigan. In January 2018 three advocacy groups, the National Health Law Program, the Kentucky Equal Justice Center, and the Southern Poverty Law Center, sued Kentucky on behalf of 15 state residents (*Stewart v. Azar*, 308 F. Supp. 3rd, 239 [US Dist. 2018]). The suit alleged that the Trump waiver aimed to "comprehensively transform" and "re-write the Medicaid Act" while bypassing Congress. The plaintiffs attacked multiple waiver provisions as "arbitrary and capricious." They claimed that CMS had violated the Administrative Procedure Act by announcing its new orientation toward Medicaid waivers via a letter to state officials rather than the formal rule-making process. The plaintiffs charged that the new waiver policy also violated the president's constitutional duty to "take care that the laws be faithfully executed"(First Am. Class Action Compl. for Declaratory and Injunctive Relief, *Stewart v. Azar*, 308 F. Supp. 3rd [US Dist. 2018] [No. 18–152 (JEB)]). The Kentucky challenge along with the Arkansas and New Hampshire suits were heard separately by Judge James Boasberg (an Obama appointee) in a district court of the DC Circuit. In a series of decisions halting implementation of three of the waivers (with the suits against Indiana and Michigan pending), Boasberg did not explicitly address whether Medicaid law permitted work requirements or other provisions. Instead, he vacated the waivers on grounds that they were likely to produce enrollment declines inconsistent with the coverage goals embedded in the Medicaid statute. He noted that the Kentucky waiver proposal had projected a substantial enrollment decline. Moreover, one study estimated that 600,000–800,000 enrollees would lose coverage if nine states with approved work-requirement waivers implemented them (Ku and Brantley 2019). As a result of Boasberg's rulings, the implementation of the work requirement waivers ground to a halt by the end of 2019. The Trump administration unsuccessfully appealed these decisions to the DC Circuit and the case might eventually land on the docket of the Supreme Court. If Trump officials ultimately prevail in the courts, it would greatly enhance the utility of waivers as a policy tool for the administrative presidency.

Meanwhile, the Trump administration announced its intention to consider state demonstration waiver proposals that would block-grant Medicaid rather than preserve it as an entitlement. Depending on their specifics, these waivers could also erode Medicaid coverage. In early 2020, CMS issued guidelines that invited states to submit block grant proposals.

The 1332 Innovation Waivers: Weakening the Guardrails

The ACA authorized states as of 2017 to propose section 1332 waivers to pursue innovative alternatives to achieving the law's goals. The Trump administration's initial use of these waivers departed from its more general sabotage efforts (Thompson, Gusmano, and Shinohara 2018). In his letter to governors in early March 2017, Secretary Price invited states to submit proposals that would slow the rate of premium growth and improve the exchange risk pools. The letter pointed to "reinsurance" as one way to accomplish this. This approach offered subsidies to insurance companies for covering people with more costly medical needs, allowing the exchanges to set lower premiums that would presumably help them attract healthier enrollees. In mid-2017, the agency approved a 1332 waiver proposal from Alaska that allowed the state to use federal funds to defray the cost of a reinsurance program. The lower premiums that resulted would reduce the tax credits that the federal government provided to exchange enrollees with incomes below 400% of the poverty line. By late 2019, 11 more states (Colorado, Delaware, Maine, Maryland, Minnesota, Montana, New Jersey, North Dakota, Oregon, Rhode Island, and Wisconsin) received CMS blessings to use reinsurance. The successful proposals came from relatively liberal states, with 8 of the 12 having voted for Hillary Clinton in 2016. We cannot explain why the Trump administration abandoned its overall strategy of sabotaging the marketplaces to buttress them through reinsurance waivers. It may be, however, that principles of federalism mattered, where the administration's declared commitment to greater state flexibility overrode its desire to undermine the exchanges.

Subsequent 1332 actions by the Trump administration were more consistent with sabotage. As noted earlier, the Obama administration had established "guardrails" for these waivers in 2015 to protect the ACA from erosion. The guardrails insisted that state alternatives provide coverage at least as comprehensive and as affordable as the ACA. They also stipulated that the waiver insure at least a comparable number of state residents and not increase the federal deficit. In October 2018, CMS issued new guidelines to the states to replace the Obama guardrails. The new guidelines changed the name of the initiatives to "State Relief and Empowerment Waivers." They prioritized access to coverage over the quality ("comprehensiveness and content") of insurance in reviewing state proposals. The guidance encouraged state proposals that would ask the federal government to subsidize enrollment in non-compliant-ACA products, such as short-term and association health plans. These plans would not necessarily cover the ACA's 10 essential health benefits or provide affordable access to care for those with preexisting conditions. They heightened the risk that healthier people would exit the exchanges to purchase cheaper, lower-quality coverage, worsening the exchange risk pools (Cohen 2018). The Obama guardrails had also insisted that the legislature and the governor sign off on a waiver proposal. The Trump administration relaxed this requirement and made it easier for a governor to submit the waiver application without specific legislative authorization.

The degree to which the new CMS guidelines would fuel flight from the ACA-compliant exchanges to lower-quality plans (what Democrats call "junk insurance") depended on state willingness to pursue such waivers. Six months later, no state had requested waivers in response to the new section 1332 guidance. Concerned by this lack of interest, CMS Administrator Verma in late April 2019 implored states to take advantage of the new waiver flexibility (Lotven 2019). Finally, Republican Governor Brian Kemp of Georgia announced in early November that his state would accept the CMS invitation. Among other things, the Georgia proposed 1332 waiver would allow individuals with incomes below 400% of poverty to use their federal tax credits to subsidize the purchase of noncompliant ACA coverage, such as short-term health plans (Cohen 2019). Whether the Georgia proposal, when submitted and formally approved, will survive a certain court challenge remained an open question as 2020 dawned.

Conclusion

Waivers have helped fuel the growth in executive branch discretion to shape who gets what in health care. The professional bureaucratic complex, consisting of state and federal officials with similar educations and work experiences, at times dominates the exercise of this discretion (e.g., as with section 1915 waivers). As demonstrated in this article, however, decisions concerning waivers can also become part and parcel of the administrative presidency and swayed more by partisan preferences. Both the Obama and Trump administrations strove to use comprehensive waivers to shape ACA implementation.

The Obama administration experienced mixed success in employing this tool. Its deployment of market-oriented demonstration waivers helped entice seven otherwise reluctant states to participate in the Medicaid expansion at all or to do so earlier than they otherwise would have. This "reluctant" waiver cohort comprised over a fifth of all Medicaid expansion states by the time Obama left office. This participatory outcome proved durable at least through the first 3 years of the Trump administration, as none of the states had withdrawn from the expansion. The Obama administration won this victory without making major concessions on work requirements, cost sharing, or partial expansions that certain states had sought. As for the 1332 waivers, the Obama administration forged guardrails that would make it difficult for states to erode the ACA through innovation proposals. But waivers hardly proved to be an elixir for the Obama administrative presidency. Most Republican-dominated states evinced little or no interest in negotiating demonstration waivers leading to Medicaid expansion. Other Obama efforts to incentivize Medicaid expansions by cutting back on waivers allowing special hospital pools for uncompensated care in nonparticipating states did not have the desired effects. Moreover, the Trump administration promptly reversed the policy. And, Trump officials moved apace to weaken the 1332 guardrails that Obama officials had established to protect the ACA from erosion.

Compared to Obama, the Trump administration has found it harder to accomplish its policy goals through waivers. Its biggest success has been encouraging the diffusion of reinsurance waivers, which have damped down premium increases and generally bolstered the exchanges. Beyond that, two of its major waiver initiatives foundered. First, despite widespread interest in work requirement waivers among conservative states and CMS willingness to approve them, the federal courts have blocked their implementation. Second, the Trump administration's weakening of Obama-era 1332 guardrails to invite states to promote cheaper noncompliant ACA insurance in their marketplaces had, with the exception of Georgia, triggered minimal state interest by the end of 2019. Of course, this portrait of the "Trump administrative presidency stymied" might over time morph into a picture of "Trump triumphant." If the courts support the Trump administration's work requirement and 1332 waiver initiatives, it would signal their approval of a highly expansive reading of pertinent statutes by the executive branch. It would raise the question of what, if any, congressional statutory limits apply to what can be done through waivers. It would enable the president to use waivers to achieve an ever broader set of goals, including program retrenchment.

■ ■ ■

Michael K. Gusmano is associate professor in the School of Public Health's Department of Health Behavior, Society, and Policy and Administration at Rutgers University. He also is a research scholar at the Hastings Center and a visiting fellow at the Nelson A. Rockefeller Institute of Government of the State University of New York. He serves as the international editor of the *Journal of Aging and Social Policy* and associate editor for *Health Economics, Policy and Law* and is on the board of editors of the *Journal of Health Politics, Policy and Law* and the editorial committee of the *Hastings Center Report*.
gusmanom@thehastingscenter.org

Frank J. Thompson is Board of Governors' Distinguished Professor of Public Affairs and Administration at Rutgers University–Newark and at the Rutgers Center for State Health Policy in New Brunswick. He has published extensively on issues of health policy, with particular attention to the impact of federalism. His most recent book (with Kenneth Wong and Barry Rabe) is *Trump, the Administrative Presidency and Federalism* (in press with the Brookings Institution). Recent publications have focused on the administrative presidency and Obamacare, Medicaid waivers for delivery system reform, and other Medicaid topics. He is a fellow of the National Academy of Public Administration.

References

CMS (Centers for Medicare and Medicaid Services). 2018. "Opportunities to Promote Work and Community Engagement among Medicaid Beneficiaries." Letter to state Medicaid directors, January 11. www.medicaid.gov/sites/default/files/federal -policy-guidance/downloads/smd18002.pdf.

Cohen, Ariel. 2017. "CMS No Longer Lists Expanding Coverage as a Goal of 1115 Waivers." Inside Health Policy, November 15. insidehealthpolicy.com/inside-cms /cms-no-longer-lists-expanding-coverage-goal-1115-waivers.

Cohen, Ariel, 2018. "CMS Shifts Focus of 1332 Waivers to Bolster Non-ACA Coverage." Inside Health Policy, October 22. insidehealthpolicy.com/daily-news/cms -shifts-focus-1332-waivers-bolster-non-aca-coverage.

Cohen, Ariel. 2019. "Georgia to Apply for ACA Waiver under New Trump Rules." Inside Health Policy, October 31. insidehealthpolicy.com/daily-news/georgia-apply -aca-waiver-under-new-trump-rules.

GAO (Government Accountability Office). 2019a. "Medicaid Demonstrations: Approvals of Major Changes Need Increased Transparency." April. www.gao.gov /assets/700/698608.pdf.

GAO (Government Accountability Office). 2019b. "Medicaid Demonstrations: Actions Need to Address Weaknesses in Oversight of Costs to Administer Work Requirements." October. www.gao.gov/assets/710/701885.pdf.

Howell, William. 2003. *Power without Persuasion*. Princeton, NJ: Princeton University Press.

Ku, Leighton, and Erin Brantley. 2019. "Medicaid Work Requirements in Nine States Could Cause 600,000 to 800,000 Adults to Lose Medicaid Coverage." Commonwealth Fund, June 21. www.commonwealthfund.org/blog/2019/medicaid-work -requirements-nine-states-could-cause-600000-800000-adults-lose-coverage.

Lewis, David. 2008. *The Politics of Presidential Appointments: Political Control and Bureaucratic Performance*. Princeton, NJ: Princeton University Press.

Lotven, Amy. 2019. "CMS RFI Seeks to Spur State Interest in Eased 1332 Waiver Criteria." Inside Health Policy, May 1. insidehealthpolicy.com/daily-news/cms-rfi -seeks-spur-states%E2%80%99-interest-eased-1332-waiver-criteria.

McDonough, John E. 2015. "The Demise of Vermont's Single-Payer Plan." *New England Journal of Medicine* 372: 1584–85.

Moynihan, Donald, Pamela Herd, and Hope Harvey. 2015. "Administrative Burden: Learning, Psychological, and Compliance Costs in Citizen-State Interactions." *Journal of Public Administration Research and Theory* 25, no. 1: 43–70.

Nathan, Richard P. 1983. *The Administrative Presidency*. New York: Wiley.

Price, Thomas E., and Seema Verma. 2017. "Letter to State Governors." US Department of Health and Human Services, March 14. www.hhs.gov/about/news/2017/03/14 /secretary-price-and-cms-administrator-verma-take-first-joint-action.html.

Rudowitz, Robin, MaryBeth Musumeci, and Cornelia Hall. 2018. "A Look at November State Data for Medicaid Work Requirements in Arkansas." Kaiser Family Foundation, December. files.kff.org/attachment/Issue-Brief-A-Look-at -November-State-Data-for-Medicaid-Work-Requirements-in-Arkansas.

Thompson, Frank J., Michael K. Gusmano, and Shugo Shinohara. 2018. "Trump and the Affordable Care Act: Congressional Repeal Efforts, Executive Federalism, and Program Durability." *Publius* 48, no. 3: 396–424.

Thompson, Frank J., Kenneth K. Wong, and Barry G. Rabe. Forthcoming. *Trump, the Administrative Presidency, and Federalism*. Washington, DC: Brookings Institution.

Verma, Seema. 2017. "Remarks by Administrator Seema Verma." National Association of Medicaid Directors fall conference, Arlington, VA, November 7. www.cms.gov /newsroom/fact-sheets/speech-remarks-administrator-seema-verma-national-associ ation-medicaid-directors-namd-2017–fall.

The Affordable Care Act in the States: Fragmented Politics, Unstable Policy

Daniel Béland
McGill University

Philip Rocco
Marquette University

Alex Waddan
University of Leicester

Abstract Many argue that the frustrated implementation of the 2010 Affordable Care Act (ACA) stems from the unprecedented level of political polarization that has surrounded the legislation. This article draws attention to the law's "institutional DNA" as a source of political struggle in the 50 states. As designed, in the context of US federalism, the law fractured authority in ways that has opened up the possibility of contestation and confusion. The successful implementation of the ACA varies not only across state lines but also across the various components of the law. In particular, opponents of the ACA have experienced their greatest successes when they could take advantage of weak preexisting policy legacies, high levels of institutional fragmentation, and negative public sentiments. As argued in this article, the fragmented patterns of health care politics in the 50 states identified in previous research have largely persisted during the Trump administration. Moreover, while Republicans were unsuccessful at repealing the legislation, the administration has taken advantage of its structural deficiencies to further weaken the legislation's capacity to expand access to affordable, quality health insurance.

Keywords Affordable Care Act, Obamacare, health care reform, federalism, states, United States

The signing ceremony of the Affordable Care Act (ACA)—the most dramatic reform of the US health care system since the creation of Medicare and Medicaid—was a moment of almost unmitigated optimism. The law, President Obama said, was an affirmation of the "core principle that everybody should have some basic security when it comes to their core health care" and an "essential truth" that "we are not a nation that scales

Journal of Health Politics, Policy and Law, Vol. 45, No. 4, August 2020
DOI 10.1215/03616878-8255565   © 2020 by Duke University Press

back its aspirations" (Stolberg and Pear 2010). Yet the law represented a series of scaled-back aspirations—an attempt to make real reforms while keeping the basic structure of American health care financing in place. Compromises with the insurance and pharmaceutical industries, as well as fiscal conservatives within the Democratic Party, resulted in a law that required many middle-income Americans to purchase insurance on confusing and glitch-laden marketplaces and that buried fiscal benefits in a tax-expenditure scheme. Before long, the Supreme Court had scaled back the effect of the law's most tangible and visible benefit, Medicaid expansion, by allowing state governments to opt out. In addition, while the US uninsurance rate fell steeply following the passage of the ACA, 13.7% of the US population remained uninsured by 2019. This represented a 4-year high, suggesting that coverage gains made under the Obama administration have begun to recede slightly under Trump (Witters 2019).

Many argue that the ACA's frustrated implementation can be explained by the unprecedented level of political polarization that has surrounded the legislation. In our book *Obamacare Wars* (Béland, Rocco, and Waddan 2016), however, we draw attention to the law's "institutional DNA" as a source of struggle. As designed, the law fractured authority in ways that opened up the possibility of contestation and confusion. The successful implementation of the ACA varied not only across state lines but also across the various components of the law. In particular, opponents of the ACA experienced their greatest successes when they could take advantage of weak preexisting policy legacies, high levels of institutional fragmentation, and negative public sentiments.

The fragmented patterns of politics we identified have largely persisted during the Trump administration. Moreover, while Republicans were unsuccessful at repealing the legislation, the administration has taken advantage of its structural deficiencies to further weaken the legislation's capacity to expand access to affordable, quality health insurance.

Insurance Exchanges

The core objective of health insurance marketplaces is to offer affordable insurance packages tied to government subsidies. Both small businesses and lower-income people ineligible for Medicaid are targeted by these insurance marketplaces (Béland, Rocco, and Waddan 2016). As the name implies, marketplaces are market-friendly institutions, which is probably why the framers of the ACA did not expect a strong Republican backlash against them at the state level. Yet this political backlash did occur, and as of 2018, only 12 jurisdictions, including DC, operated state-based marketplaces. In contrast, federally facilitated marketplaces were in place in 34 states. The last 5 states operated a state-based marketplace "using a federal platform" (Forsberg 2018: 2). This means that only a small minority of states elected to run their own health insurance marketplaces. This situation forced the federal government to spend much effort and money setting up marketplaces, a situation that further complicated the implementation of the ACA (Béland, Rocco, and Waddan 2016). Yet, at least the federal government could act on its own in this component of the ACA, a situation that contrasts with Medicaid expansion, which requires states to take the lead. Simultaneously, the extremely favorable fiscal incentives associated with Medicaid expansion nudged a greater number of states to participate in this other key component of the reform. Moreover, in contrast with other aspects of the law, outside of post-Romneycare Massachusetts, health insurance marketplaces appeared as a novelty states had no experience dealing with. Finally, because of their high public profile and their direct link with the controversial and widely debated "individual mandate," health insurance marketplaces offered ACA opponents in the states an opportunity to demonstrate their opposition to the law by refusing to set up their own exchanges (Béland, Rocco, and Waddan 2016).

A fascinating aspect of the limited adoption of "homemade" marketplaces by the states is the fact that opposition to this policy tool emerged only after the ACA's enactment (Jones, Bradley, and Oberlander 2014). This is because, as suggested above, marketplaces are inspired by Romneycare and market-friendly policy ideas that Republicans had long embraced. Yet, once they became part of the ACA, exchanges suffered from "guilt by association," as many GOP-governed states rejected the reform as a block (Jones, Bradley, and Oberlander 2014). Conversely, the widely publicized problems experienced by some health insurance marketplaces have been used to discredit the ACA as a whole, even if these exchanges are only one component of it (Altman 2016).

Here a double ideological simplification is taking place. First, the problems witnessed in some states are used to promote the idea that all state exchanges are dysfunctional. Second, the concept of the ACA as a whole is reduced to the system of health insurance marketplaces and to the "individual mandate" so central to the conservative rhetoric against the ACA. While the individual mandate was envisioned as an essential means of avoiding adverse selection in the marketplaces, it remained enduringly unpopular. This may explain why, of all the potential repeal-and-replace plans congressional Republicans introduced in 2017, the proposal to eliminate the individual mandate came closest to passing on its own, losing by a one-vote margin in the Senate (Béland, Rocco, and Waddan 2019). While it would never receive a public vote, the penalty for the individual mandate was later zeroed out by Republicans in omnibus tax overhaul legislation, setting the stage for new litigation on the constitutionality of the ACA in *Texas v. United States* (No. 19–10011, 5th Cir. 2019). Thus, while the marketplaces remained in place, the zeroing out of the mandate reveals how the sheer complexity of the ACA obscures the link between the law's popular and unpopular components (Altman 2016; on obfuscation, see Pierson 1994).

For the time being, like the ACA itself, health insurance marketplaces are here to stay, in part because they have created their own policy legacies over time. Interestingly, states that decided to implement their own marketplaces witness lower insurance premiums on average than do states that decided to let the federal government do all the work (Alberts and Cousart 2017; Hall and McCue 2018). This reality has a key political implication: the decision of many states to pass on the opportunity to set up their own exchanges has been detrimental to the residents of these states while contributing directly to weakening public support for the ACA. This is because exchanges, especially those that do not perform well, remain to the foreground of the ideological struggles over the ACA. Such a situation sharply contrasts with the situation prevailing in the field of health insurance regulation, where successful cooperation between the federal government and the states has been the norm rather than the exception (Béland, Rocco, and Waddan 2016).

Medicaid Expansion

The Supreme Court's decision in June 2012, which gave states a genuine choice about whether to join the Medicaid expansion, effectively changed the policy design of the ACA and made this aspect of the law a subject of ongoing political contestation. Nearly 6 years after the expansion came into effect, 14 states still refused to embrace the federal dollars on offer and extend health insurance to some of the poorest people in the state. Simultaneously, some states have sought to use the section 1115 waiver process to get leeway from the Trump administration to make Medicaid eligibility conditional on requirements in ways that the ACA's framers never intended. Hence, the Medicaid expansion has seen the noisiest ongoing politics—and this is not a symbolic politics, put on simply for performance, but is a politics where the results have grave real-world consequences.

Deeper policy legacies and lower levels of institutional fragmentation have helped encourage states to expand Medicaid. Unlike with the insurance exchanges, which asked states if they wanted to engage in building new institutions, all states already had experience with Medicaid. Certainly more states had joined the expansion by the end of Obama's time in office than had set up their own insurance exchange. Yet, reflecting existing policy trajectories, those states with more generous existing eligibility criteria were more likely to join the expansion than those with "stingier" requirements (Morone 2012).

Developments on a state-by-state level also hinged on institutional arrangements within states. One recurring, if not typical, occurrence was a battle between a state's governor and its legislature. Notably, some red states had joined the expansion in circumstances where the state's governor had taken control of the process and overridden opposition from the state legislature. In Ohio, Governor John Kasich used arcane rules to bypass the legislature, and in Arizona, Governor Jan Brewer, no friend to the Obama administration, effectively leveraged her powers to force the legislature to agree to join the expansion. In Florida, in contrast, the legislature was not to be bypassed, and Governor Rick Scott's flirtation with the idea of joining the expansion was squashed, and in Maine, Republican governor Paul LePage used his power to veto bills passed by the Democratic legislature to expand the state's Medicaid program.

Other more recent examples have reinforced the importance of the willingness and capacity of a governor to wield executive power to push through the expansion. Louisiana was the first, and remains the only, Deep South state to adopt the expansion following the election of Democrat John Bel Edwards to the governorship. On his second day in office Edwards issued an executive order to set the expansion process in motion (Miller 2016), despite the fact that the GOP retained comfortable control of both chambers of the state legislature. By February 2017, over 400,000 people had enrolled and the state's uninsured rate had fallen from 21.7% in 2013 to 12.5% (Louisiana Department of Health 2017). Meanwhile in Virginia, Democratic governor Terry McAuliffe was thwarted in his efforts to expand the state's Medicaid program by the state legislature, despite 4 years of trying. In the end, his successor, Democratic governor Ralph Northam, was able to sign an expansion into law in June 2018 after Democrats gained several seats in the state's House of Delegates elections in 2017 (Goodnough 2018). This was also predicted to cover up to 400,000 people. In contrast, in Kansas in 2017, both chambers of the Republican-controlled legislature voted to accept the expansion, if with caveats, but Governor Sam Brownback vetoed that move.

In addition to policy legacies and institutional fragmentation, public sentiments are a crucial factor that has shaped ACA politics. We define public sentiments as *"issue salience* and *public support"* for policy initiatives (Béland, Rocco, and Waddan 2016: 33; on public sentiments, see also Campbell 2004). Since 2017, the question of public support has been tested explicitly on Medicaid, as several states have seen referenda on the matter. In 2017, in Maine 59% of voters approved expanding the state's Medicaid program, though Governor Le Page yet again stood in defiance. Finally, in January 2019, new Democratic governor Janet Mills called for the expansion to be implemented.

One analysis of the votes cast in Maine, however, suggested that this was not necessarily a pattern that would be widely repeated. Matsa and Miller (2019) tentatively concluded that, if a similar exercise in direct democracy were conducted in the 18 states that had not at that point expanded their Medicaid program, only 5 would have a pro-expansion majority.[1] Yet, showing broader support, or at least more mobilized support, than implied in that model, in November 2018 three red states, Idaho, Nebraska, and Utah, voted to expand their Medicaid programs with 61%, 53%, and 54% of voters, respectively, supporting expansion (Kliff 2018).[2] Further, Clinton and Sances (2018: 183) suggest some, if quite modest, increase in political participation resulting from the expansion "concentrated among potential beneficiaries" (see also Michener 2017)

The story told so far is suggestive of some momentum, if very halting and far from comprehensive, edging toward an expansion of the expansion. But even such a heavily qualified narrative is too one-dimensional. No state has repealed its expansion outright, even in cases where the expansion was pushed through in red-leaning states by a Democrat governor who was then succeeded by a conservative Republican. Perhaps most starkly, in Kentucky in 2015, Republican Matt Bevin campaigned on repealing the Medicaid expansion pushed through by his Democratic predecessor Steve Beshear.[3] In fact, even before Election Day, Bevin, presenting himself as a Tea Party conservative, was walking back that commitment, given the ramifications of taking away the coverage of about 400,000 of the state's population (Pradhan and Demko 2015). Yet, the state has aggressively pursued the application of work requirements in a manner that undermines key principles of the ACA.

1. This was a hypothetical analysis assuming that all the states could conduct a referendum, which was not the case. The analysis was conducted before Virginia expanded its program.
2. Matsa and Miller's (2019) model predicted that Utah would support expansion but that Idaho and Nebraska would not.
3. Beshear relied on executive authority to expand Medicaid in Kentucky, though at the time the Democrats also controlled the state House.

One of the novel features of the ACA's version of expansion, in contrast to the existing Medicaid rules, was that it set out to determine eligibility simply according to income, at least up to its floor of 138% of the poverty level, without additional judgment on the "moral worthiness" of beneficiaries. In addition, the Obama administration made it clear that it was unwilling to allow states much discretion to veer from that unconditional standard. For example, Indiana was allowed to introduce a monthly copayment for Medicaid recipients, but this was limited to a minimum of $1 rather than the $3 requested by the state (Samuels 2016). In addition, work requirements were not permitted. The Trump administration, however, has taken quite a different path in allowing states to employ section 1115 waivers to impose tougher conditions for people to qualify for access to the expanded program.[4]

In this context, efforts to roll back statewide expansions have taken the form of applying work requirements and other conditions to encourage "personal responsibility" rather than simple repeal. Arkansas was the first state to forcefully implement work-reporting requirements, and between June 2018 and January 2019, 18,000 people had lost their entitlement to Medicaid because of failing to meet the new standards (Scheneider 2019). To counter these actions, advocates of more unconditional Medicaid expansion turned to a tactic aggressively and repeatedly used by the ACA's opponents by challenging these moves in court. This resulted in Arkansas and Kentucky having their actions suspended for conflicting with the Administrative Procedure Act (Schneider 2019). Nevertheless, with Trump's Department of Health and Human Services willing to grant states considerable autonomy in devising their Medicaid expansion programs, this type of policy redesign of the original ACA is likely to feature across a number of states.

Overall, in the years since it was implemented, the Medicaid expansion has become a source of both health and economic security, covering nearly 12.7 million newly eligible Americans by 2017 (Kaiser Family Foundation, n.d.). Even since then, the number of states participating in one form or another of Medicaid expansion has crept up, yet policy routes taken across states remain quite diverse. As described by Richardson (2019: 448), we should acknowledge that there are effectively "three Medicaid policy

---

4. Some nonexpansion states have also sought waivers to apply work requirements to the pre-ACA Medicaid population. Two such states, Alabama and Mississippi, have adult Medicaid eligibility levels set at 18% and 26% of the federal poverty level, respectively, meaning that an adult working even part-time would possibly become ineligible for Medicaid (Garfield et al. 2019: 5).

trajectories in the states—full ACA expansion, section 1115 waivers with personal responsibility features, and nonexpansion states with limited Medicaid coverage for able adults."

Regulatory Reforms

While not as salient as the exchanges or the Medicaid expansion, the ACA's suite of regulatory reforms has been a political and policy backbone for the law. These include the law's prohibition on preexisting condition exclusions, its guaranteed-issue requirement, and its community-rating provisions, as well as a number of other consumer protections aimed at both expanding access to insurance regardless of health status and mandating essential health benefits.

The politics of implementing the ACA's regulatory reforms at the state level have differed from the insurance exchanges and the Medicaid expansion in three important ways. First, unlike the exchanges, the ACA's regulatory reforms built on preexisting policy legacies in the states. To be sure, few if any states maintained the elaborate consumer protections developed by the ACA, but most had laid down policy frameworks on consumer protection, review of insurer rates, and medical loss ratios on which the ACA's new regulations could be built. Second, the ACA's regulatory reforms employed a less fragmented set of consent procedures than other components of the law (see also Fahey 2014). For example, whereas the creation of insurance exchanges and the expansion of Medicaid generally required some combination of gubernatorial and legislative action, many states came into compliance with the ACA's early market reforms (e.g., the ban on preexisting condition exclusions) without any formal legislative or regulatory action. Rather, insurance commissioners issued subregulatory guidance or indicated that they were reviewing insurance policies in accordance with the ACA's new standards (Béland, Rocco, and Waddan 2016: 133–35). Those who wished to block them at the state level were forced to use the legislative process to claw back consumer protections. But such actions were not likely to produce political rewards. While the regulatory reforms were among the more popular of the ACA's provisions, they were not as politically salient as either the exchanges or the Medicaid expansion.

In one sense, the speedy implementation of regulatory reforms has been a source of political stability for the ACA. While the law's protections for individuals with preexisting conditions were not initially salient, the threat of repeal that followed Republicans' 2016 election victory helped enhance their visibility and public approval, even as other dimensions of the law remained controversial (Peterson 2018). While less visible than the consumer protections, the ACA's medical loss ratio reforms delivered rebates to consumers as insurers raised rates and profits increased (Hall and McCue 2019). Moreover, even as the Trump administration has sought to undermine the ACA in other ways, it has generally enforced existing consumer protections, even threatening to take over enforcement in states that have attempted to skirt compliance (Pear 2018).

Yet, as our earlier research noted, it is not enough to analyze the formal stability of these reforms (Béland, Rocco, and Waddan 2016: 150–52). Rather, retrenchment can occur in the absence of formal repeal, through gradual institutional changes (Hacker, Pierson, and Thelen 2015). In the case of the ACA's regulatory reforms, gradual change occurred not through state action but through the Trump administration's conversion of federal regulations. Five examples stand out.

First, the Trump administration expanded the availability of short-term limited-duration insurance, which the Obama administration determined was adversely affecting risk pools in individual markets (Keith 2018b). Whereas the ACA's medical loss ratio rule requires insurers to spend at least 80% of their premiums on delivering services to customers, the top three issuers of short-term insurance collectively spent less than 43.8% (Livingston 2019). Second, a 2018 labor department rule significantly relaxed the regulation of association health plans, despite objections from state insurance regulators and evidence that it would lead to premium increases and higher levels of uninsurance (Keith 2018a). Third, under rules that will become effective in 2020, the Trump administration is allowing states to alter requirements on essential health benefits and diminish individual-market medical loss ratios (Keith 2018c). Fourth, the Trump administration has proposed rules that will loosen the ACA's prohibitions on language-, sex-, and disability-based discrimination (Keith 2019). Finally, the Trump administration refused to intervene to defend the ACA against new constitutional challenges posed by Judge Reed O'Connor's sweeping decision in *Texas v. United States* (No. 4:18–cv-167–O, N.D. Tex., 2018), which held that the entire ACA is unconstitutional. While the Fifth Circuit Court of Appeals upheld O'Connor's decision on the individual mandate, it punted on the issue of severability — effectively asking O'Connor to "parse through" the law with a "finer-toothed comb" to determine which sections may be severable from the individual mandate.

States' responses to policy changes brought about by the Trump administration vary significantly. While many states came into compliance with the ACA without extensive legislative or gubernatorial involvement, protecting consumers from new substandard plans may take a greater level of positive action. As Giovanelli, Lucia, and Corlette (2018) highlight, fewer than half of the states set stricter limits on short-term, limited-duration insurance than the federal government. At present, fewer than five states have statutes that specifically enshrine essential health benefits, prohibit annual or lifetime limits on benefits, require preventive services without cost sharing, and incorporate the ACA's nondiscrimination provisions (Corlette and Curran 2019).

States are also underprepared for the existential threat to the ACA posed by *Texas v. United States.* If the district court's decision is ultimately upheld, numerous states will find themselves without statutory support for the ACA's regulatory reforms. While less fragmented consent procedures helped with implementation of these reforms, fewer than half the states have enacted legislation specifically enshrining community ratings, guaranteed issue, and bans on preexisting condition exclusion (Corlette and Curran 2019). If the ACA is ultimately struck down, state lawmakers will obviously experience political pressure to reauthorize these protections. Nevertheless, that will require a greater degree of institutional action than was required when the ACA was initially implemented. Most important, in the absence of federal payments, state fiscal capacities will be inadequate to subsidize coverage on the marketplaces, rendering them dysfunctional. In short, the judicial invalidation of the ACA would result in a fair amount of chaos and confusion in state insurance regulations.

Conclusion

There are few easy historical parallels to the postenactment life of the ACA. Enacted on a party-line vote and in a context of intense polarization, its implementation could not be expected to resemble that of Medicare, or even of Medicaid, half a century earlier. Nor does the ACA's postenactment politics resemble that of the Medicare Catastrophic Coverage Act, which Congress quickly repealed after enactment (Peterson 2018). Rather, the ACA's fragmented structure has produced multiple political dynamics across various dimensions of the law. Indeed, the turbulence that has defined policy making in the Trump era, variations policy legacies, institutional fragmentation, and public sentiments have continued to matter.

While the ACA continues to display multiple political dynamics, the Trump administration's assault on the law has had an effect on how these dynamics play out. Although the law's regulatory reforms were quickly implemented through subregulatory guidance and consultation, few states have put in place legislation to preserve them should the law be struck down in *Texas v. United States*. Procedural tools like waivers, which helped promote Medicaid expansion during the Obama years, have been used by the Trump administration as a means of policy retrenchment, both of Medicaid expansion and of benefits created prior to the passage of the ACA. Individual marketplaces created by state governments may be resilient, even if constitutional challenges to the law succeed. Yet the fact that few states created these marketplaces in the first place remains a source of vulnerability for the endurance of the law.

For the reader interested in a neat description of "where we are now," none of these conclusions will be satisfactory. Nor is it wise to make broad pronouncements about the future of the ACA. Even so, there are clear lessons here for those who design and implement major reforms. In environments of intense political contestation, designing policy with weak legacies and fragmented institutional designs opens up vulnerabilities that are not easily addressed with traditional policy tools. Intergovernmental grants, consultation procedures, and regulatory clarity still matter, of course. However, when intense political conflict persists after enactment—and especially when implementation is decentralized—the task of political persuasion and coalition building remains. No reform—and certainly not one as significant as the ACA—has ever been self-implementing.

▪ ▪ ▪

Daniel Béland is director of the McGill Institute for the Study of Canada and James McGill Professor in the Department of Political Science at McGill University in Montreal. A student of social and fiscal policy, he has published more than 15 books and 140 articles in peer-reviewed journals such as *Governance, Health Policy, Journal of Public Policy, Journal of Social Policy*, and *Publius*. Recent books include *An Advanced Introduction to Social Policy* (2016; with Rianne Mahon) and *Obamacare Wars: Federalism, State Politics, and the Affordable Care Act* (2016; with Philip Rocco and Alex Waddan).
daniel.beland@mcgill.ca

Philip Rocco is assistant professor of political science at Marquette University. He is the coauthor of *Obamacare Wars: Federalism, State Politics, and the Affordable Care Act* (2016) and coeditor of *American Political Development and the Trump Presidency* (forthcoming). He has published in, among other venues, *Health Affairs, Journal of Health Politics, Policy and Law, Political Science Quarterly, Publius, Forum*, and *Journal of Public Policy*. He is working on a book manuscript titled *Madison's Engineers: How Policy Science Remade Federalism*.

Alex Waddan is associate professor at the University of Leicester. He is the author or coauthor of five books, including *Obamacare Wars: Federalism, State Politics, and the Affordable Care Act* (2016) and, most recently, *The American Right after Reagan* (2019). He has also published numerous book chapters and journal articles, including pieces in *Political Science Quarterly, Policy Studies Journal, Political Studies,* and the *Journal of Social Policy.* He is currently working on a project looking at the politics of health care financing in the United States and the United Kingdom.

References

Alberts, Corinne, and Christina Cousart. 2017. "Unpacking the State-Based Market-places." National Academy for State Health Policy, August 7. nashp.org/unpacking -the-state-based-marketplaces/.

Altman, Drew. 2016. "ACA Marketplace Problems in Context (and Why They Don't Mean Obamacare Is 'Failing')." *Wall Street Journal,* August 29. blogs.wsj.com /washwire/2016/08/29/the-aca-marketplace-problems-in-context-and-why-they-dont -mean-obamacare-is-failing/.

Béland, Daniel, Philip Rocco, and Alex Waddan. 2016. *Obamacare Wars: Federalism, State Politics, and the Affordable Care Act.* Lawrence: University Press of Kansas.

Béland, Daniel, Philip Rocco, and Alex Waddan. 2019. "Policy Feedback and the Politics of the Affordable Care Act." *Policy Studies Journal* 47, no. 2: 395–422.

Campbell, John L. 2004. *Institutional Change and Globalization.* Princeton, NJ: Princeton University Press.

Clinton, Joshua, and Michael Sances. 2018. "The Politics of Policy: The Initial Mass Political Effects of Medicaid Expansion in the States." *American Political Science Review* 112, no. 1: 167–85.

Corlette, Sabrina, and Emily Curran. 2019. "Can States Fill the Gap if the Federal Government Overturns Preexisting Condition Protections?" Commonwealth Fund, May 7. www.commonwealthfund.org/blog/2019/can-states-fill-gap-preexisting -condition-protections.

Fahey, Bridget. 2014. "Consent Procedures and American Federalism." *Harvard Law Review* 128, no. 6: 1561–1629.

Forsberg, Vanessa C. 2018. "Overview of Health Insurance Exchanges." Congressional Research Service, June 20. fas.org/sgp/crs/misc/R44065.pdf.

Garfield, Rachel, Robin Rudowitz, Kendal Orgera, and Anthony Domico. 2019. "Understanding the Intersection of Medicaid and Work: What Does the Data Say?" Kaiser Family Foundation, August. files.kff.org/attachment/Issue-Brief-Under standing-the-Intersection-of-Medicaid-and-Work-What-Does-the-Data-Say.

Giovanelli, Justin, Kevin Lucia, and Sabrina Corlette. 2018. "To Understand How Consumers Are Faring in the Individual Health Insurance Markets, Watch the States."

Commonwealth Fund, July 18. www.commonwealthfund.org/blog/2018/understand
-how-consumers-are-faring-individual-health-insurance-markets-watch-states.

Goodnough, Abby. 2018. "After Years of Trying, Virginia Finally Will Expand
Medicaid." *New York Times*, May 30. www.nytimes.com/2018/05/30/health
/medicaid-expansion-virginia.html.

Hacker, Jacob S., Paul Pierson, and Kathleen Thelen. 2015. "Drift and Conversion:
Hidden Faces of Institutional Change." In *Advances in Comparative-Historical
Analysis*, edited by James Mahoney and Kathleen Thelen, 180–208. Cambridge:
Cambridge University Press.

Hall, Mark A., and Michael J. McCue. 2018. "Health Insurance Markets Perform
Better in States That Run Their Own Marketplaces." Commonwealth Fund,
March 7. www.commonwealthfund.org/blog/2018/health-insurance-markets-perform
-better-states-run-their-own-marketplaces.

Hall, Mark A., and Michael J. McCue. 2019. "How the ACA's Medical Loss Ratio Rule
Protects Consumers and Insurers against Ongoing Uncertainty." Commonwealth
Fund, July 2. www.commonwealthfund.org/publications/issue-briefs/2019/jul
/how-aca-medical-loss-ratio-rule-protects-consumers-insurers.

Jones, David K., Katharine W. V. Bradley, and Jonathan Oberlander. 2014. "Pascal's
Wager: Health Insurance Exchanges, Obamacare, and the Republican Dilemma,"
Journal of Health Politics, Policy and Law 39, no. 1: 97–137.

Kaiser Family Foundation. n.d. "Medicaid Expansion Enrollment." www.kff.org
/health-reform/state-indicator/medicaid-expansion-enrollment/ (accessed February
7, 2020).

Keith, Katie. 2018a. "Final Rule Rapidly Eases Restrictions on Non-ACA-Compliant
Association Health Plans." *Health Affairs Blog*, June 21. www.healthaffairs.org/do
/10.1377/hblog20180621.671483/full/.

Keith, Katie. 2018b. "The Short-Term, Limited-Duration Coverage Final Rule: The
Background, the Content, and What Could Come Next." *Health Affairs Blog*,
August 1. www.healthaffairs.org/do/10.1377/hblog20180801.169759/full/.

Keith, Katie. 2018c. "Unpacking the Final 2019 Payment Notice (Part 1)." *Health
Affairs Blog*, April 10. www.healthaffairs.org/do/10.1377/hblog20180410.631773
/full/.

Keith, Katie. 2019. "HHS Proposes to Strip Gender Identity, Language Access Protections from ACA Anti-discrimination Rule." *Health Affairs Blog*, May 25. www
.healthaffairs.org/do/10.1377/hblog20190525.831858/full/.

Kliff, Sarah. 2018. "Idaho, Nebraska, and Utah Vote to Expand Medicaid." *Vox*,
November 7. www.vox.com/2018/11/7/18055848/medicaid-expansion-idaho
-nebraska-utah.

Livingston, Shelby. 2019. "Short-Term Health Plans Spend Little on Medical Care."
Modern Healthcare, August 6. www.modernhealthcare.com/insurance/short-term
-health-plans-spend-little-medical-care.

Louisiana Department of Health. 2017. "Medicaid Expansion Enrollment Increases to
400,635; Uninsured Rate Drops." February 16. ldh.la.gov/index.cfm/newsroom
/detail/4169.

Matsa, David, and Amalia Miller. 2019. "Who Votes for Medicaid Expansion? Lessons from Maine's 2017 Referendum." *Journal of Health Politics, Policy and Law* 44, no. 4: 563–88.

Michener, Jamila. 2017. "People, Places, Power: Medicaid Policy Concentration and Local Political Participation." *Journal of Health Politics, Policy and Law* 42, no. 5: 865–900.

Miller, Andy. 2016. "Will Louisiana's Medicaid Expansion Provide a Model for Other States?" *Georgia Health News*, June 20. www.georgiahealthnews.com/2016/06 /louisianas-medicaid-expansion-provide-model-states/.

Morone, James. 2012. "Seven Consequences of the Health Care Ruling." *New York Times*, June 28. campaignstops.blogs.nytimes.com/2012/06/28/seven-consequences -of-the-health-care-ruling/.

Pear, Robert. 2018. "Trump Administration Blocks Idaho's Plan to Circumvent Health Law." *New York Times*, March 8. www.nytimes.com/2018/03/08/us/politics/idaho -affordable-care-act-trump-administration.html.

Peterson, Mark A. 2018. "Reversing Course on Obamacare: Why Not Another Medicare Catastrophic?" *Journal of Health Politics, Policy and Law* 43, no. 4: 605–50.

Pierson, Paul. 1994. *Dismantling the Welfare State? Reagan, Thatcher, and the Politics of Retrenchment*. Cambridge: Cambridge University Press.

Pradhan, Rachana, and Paul Demko. 2015. "Kentucky Health Law Repeal: Not So Fast." Politico, November 4. www.politico.com/story/2015/11/kentucky-health -law-repeal-not-so-fast-215513.

Richardson, Lilliard. 2019. "Medicaid Expansion during the Trump Presidency: The Role of Executive Waivers, State Ballot Measures, and Attorney General Lawsuits in Shaping Intergovernmental Relations." *Publius* 49, no. 3: 437–64.

Samuels, Alana. 2016. "Indiana's Medicaid Experiment May Reveal Obamacare's Future." *Atlantic*, December 21. www.theatlantic.com/business/archive/2016/12 /medicaid-and-mike-pence/511262/.

Schneider, Andy. 2019. "Judge Blocks Arkansas and Kentucky Medicaid Work Requirement Waivers: What Does This Decision Mean for Other States?" Center for Children and Families, Georgetown University Health Policy Institute, March 28. ccf.georgetown.edu/2019/03/28/judge-blocks-arkansas-and-kentucky-medicaid -work-requirement-waivers/.

Stolberg, Sheryl Gay, and Robert Pear. 2010. "Obama Signs Health Care Overhaul into Law." *New York Times*, March 23. www.nytimes.com/2010/03/24/health/policy /24health.html/.

Witters, Dan. 2019. "US Uninsured Rate Rises to Four-Year High." Gallup, January 23. news.gallup.com/poll/246134/uninsured-rate-rises-four-year-high.aspx.

States, Federalism, and Medicaid

Have the ACA's Exchanges Succeeded? It's Complicated

David K. Jones
Sarah H. Gordon
Nicole Huberfeld
Boston University

Abstract The fight over health insurance exchanges epitomizes the rapid evolution of health reform politics in the decade since the passage of the Affordable Care Act (ACA). The ACA's drafters did not expect the exchanges to be contentious because they would expand private insurance coverage to low- and middle-income individuals who were increasingly unable to obtain employer-sponsored health insurance. Instead, exchanges became one of the primary fronts in the war over Obamacare. Have the exchanges been successful? The answer is not straightforward and requires a historical perspective through a federalism lens. What the ACA has accomplished has depended largely on whether states were invested in or resistant to implementation, as well as individual decisions by state leaders working with federal officials. Our account demonstrates that the states that have engaged with the ACA most consistently appear to have experienced greater exchange-related success. But each aspect of states' engagement with or resistance to the ACA must be counted to fully paint this picture, with significant variation among states. This variation should give pause to those considering next steps in health reform, because state variation can mean innovation and improvement but also lack of coverage, disparities, and diminished access to care.

Keywords Affordable Care Act, health insurance exchanges, federalism

The fight over health insurance exchanges epitomizes the rapid evolution of health reform politics in the decade since the passage of the Affordable Care Act (ACA). The ACA's drafters did not expect the exchanges to be contentious but, rather, saw them as "a conservative means to a liberal end" because they would expand private insurance coverage to low and middle income individuals who were increasingly unable to obtain employer-

Journal of Health Politics, Policy and Law, Vol. 45, No. 4, August 2020
DOI 10.1215/03616878-8255577   © 2020 by Duke University Press

sponsored health insurance (Jones, Bradley, and Oberlander 2014: 103). The exchanges were supposed to be set up by states to facilitate competition among commercial insurers by stimulating the individual and small group insurance markets. Instead, exchanges became one of the primary fronts in the war over Obamacare.

Most of the individual elements of the exchanges—insurance regulation and consumer protections, pooling the uninsured together to give them greater purchasing power, income-related subsidies to help people with modest incomes afford coverage, a standard benefit package, and choice among private insurance plans—were not controversial.[1] Versions of these ideas had been included in health reform proposals by prominent Republicans such as Richard Nixon, George H. W. Bush, Mitt Romney, and Paul Ryan. Yet, the Obama administration faced a surprising degree of resistance, namely, from Republican leaders, when it came time to implement the exchanges.

Have the exchanges been successful? The answer is not straightforward and requires a historical perspective through a federalism lens. What the ACA has accomplished has depended largely on whether states were invested in or resistant to implementation, as well as individual decisions by state leaders working with federal officials. Cross-state comparisons show adopting a suite of policies designed to reduce the uninsured rate— such as investing in outreach, establishing a state-based exchange, and Medicaid expansion—resulted in stronger insurance markets. But these options rely heavily on local political will.

We begin by highlighting how and why states made key decisions; then we discuss the metrics that should be used to evaluate the impact of the exchanges. These two sections lead to the conclusion that the exchanges have been least impactful in the states that used the exchange as an opportunity to oppose the law's existence and most successful where leaders cooperated with the Obama administration—or at least got out of the way. We conclude by considering the future of the exchanges in the next chapter of health reform.

---

1. In addition, new federal rules established consumer protections such as essential health benefits that all qualified health plans (QHPs) must cover to be sold on an exchange, including services commonly excluded in the pre-ACA individual market, such as maternity care, mental health care, and pediatric dental services. QHPs also could not impose annual or lifetime limits or exclude those with preexisting conditions. Plans were to be kept affordable through community rating, a 3:1 rating band, cost-sharing reductions, and premium tax credits that fluctuate based on individual income and the price of benchmark plans. Plans were also standardized across four "metal" tiers of actuarial value.

Fifty Reenactments of the ACA Fight

The Obama administration's central goal for the ACA was to move toward universal coverage with at least some bipartisan support. Developments at the state level suggested that exchanges were an important component of a bipartisan strategy to achieving that goal. Ed Haislmaier (2006) of the Heritage Foundation said of the 2006 Massachusetts health reform—largely constructed around the first statewide insurance exchange—that governors and legislators would be "well advised to consider this basic model as a framework for health care reform in their own states." Utah, one of the most conservative states in the country, followed this blueprint and passed Utah H.B. 188 in 2009 to create an exchange for small businesses, with 96.3% of Republicans voting in favor. Polling suggested that more than half of Republicans supported the idea of providing tax credits to help people buy insurance in a state-based exchange (KFF 2010). Yet, by the time open enrollment began for the ACA in October 2013, 34 states had rejected control of their exchange.

For many reasons, giving states a major role in the creation of exchanges seemed like a good idea, including that the ACA might not have been enacted any other way. When the bill that ultimately became the law passed the Senate on December 24, 2009, Democrats had exactly 60 seats, meaning they could not spare a single vote and still overcome the threat of a Republican filibuster. Relying on the joint federal/state governance of federalism gave conservative Democrats a response to anyone describing the bill as a national government takeover. However, Scott Brown's election in Massachusetts a few weeks later meant that Democrats had lost their filibuster-proof majority, and passing the bill in December with state-based exchanges was the only path to enacting health reform.

Tim Jost was correct when he warned in 2009 that giving states a prominent role in implementation would open the door to 50 reenactments in state capitals of the fight Congress had just experienced (see Jost 2010). Federalism was a political pressure-release valve that made enactment possible but also dramatically complicated the politics of implementation. The law's drafters assumed that virtually every state would adopt at least a bare minimum approach to implementing its own exchange and that blue states would use their flexibility to innovate beyond the ACA. Initially, conservatives seemed to see things the same way: in 2010, 49 states began planning for a state-based exchange, including applying for and receiving $1 million federal planning grants and running local stakeholder engagement processes (Jones 2017).

Immediate Complications in Implementation

The 2010 election was the first milestone in the fight over the exchanges and the ACA's implementation. The growing Tea Party movement focused on gubernatorial and state legislative races, successfully turning blue states red and making red states redder, shifts that signaled ACA implementation might be tested. But even then, it would have been difficult to predict the intensity of opposition that would soon be leveled against the ACA and the assumption that states would want to run their own exchanges. Yet, despite the common narrative of Republicans opposing President Obama, the main partisan split in many states was not between Republicans and Democrats but within the Republican Party (Jones, Bradley, and Oberlander 2014).

Kansas offers a dramatic example of the Republican evolution. The outgoing governor was a Democrat, whose administration applied for a $31.5 million grant to be an innovator state in developing an exchange (Jones 2017). By the time the Department of Health and Human Services (HHS) considered the state's grant application in late 2010, Republican Sam Brownback had been elected governor but had not yet taken office. Brownback vehemently opposed the ACA's passage as a US Senator, and HHS wanted assurance that if they awarded Kansas the money, he would not get in the way. Governor Brownback promised HHS that Kansas would implement the ACA and be a lead exchange development state (Jones 2017).

Governor Brownback spent the first half of 2011 defending his decision to conservative groups, who felt betrayed by his cooperation with the Obama administration. He argued that, although he supported the lawsuit challenging its constitutionality, the ACA was still the law of the land. Taking money from the Obama administration was a subversive act to implement Obamacare "the Kansas way." Tea Party activists in his state and across the country disagreed. In August 2011, Governor Brownback's chief of staff and nearly a dozen Republican legislators from Kansas attended the annual meeting of the American Legislative Exchange Council (ALEC) in which Ed Haislmaier—who had described Governor Romney's law in Massachusetts as a blueprint for states to follow just five years earlier—argued that the exchanges were a frontline for opposing Obamacare. He called for "house by house, floor by floor, room by room combat" on Obamacare (Mooney 2011). Days later, Governor Brownback announced he was rejecting the HHS grant and would not build an exchange.

The year 2012 was similarly tumultuous in the fight over health insurance exchanges across the country. Some Republicans signaled they were open to creating a state-run marketplace but preferred to wait until the Supreme Court ruled in *NFIB v. Sebelius*. They did not want to undermine the lawsuit that many of them had supported and did not want to devote resources to implementing a law that they hoped would be invalidated. The Court's June 28 decision upholding the constitutionality of the individual mandate came one day before HHS's deadline for states to apply for the major grant to build information technology infrastructure in time for the start of open enrollment in October 2013. The Obama administration moved the deadline back to November, hoping that more states would pursue an exchange. But leaders in red states decided to wait until after the 2012 election, hoping Mitt Romney would be elected and follow through with his promise to undo the ACA. By the time election occurred, many leaders felt it was too late or refused to implement exchanges as an act of resistance galvanized by the Court's rendering Medicaid expansion optional. For most, the decision to delay had become a de facto decision to default to the federal exchange (Jones 2017).

Who Gets to Decide?

In many states the decision over whether or not to create an exchange came down to a fight over who decides. Seemingly mundane features of institutional design shaped the power dynamics between key players. For example, the New Mexico legislature meets for only 2 months every year and must focus in even-numbered years on the budget and bills introduced by the governor. Though states had more than 3 years to set up an exchange, the New Mexico legislature effectively had only brief windows in 2011 and 2013 to make this decision. New Mexico passed enabling legislation in March 2013, but the first decision of the newly created exchange oversight board was to default to the federal website because no time remained to develop state-specific technology.

Similarly, 10 states have insurance commissioners that are independently elected rather than appointed by the governor (Morton 2013). Mississippi's insurance commissioner, Mike Chaney, did not support the ACA but believed Mississippi would be in a better position if its exchange was regulated at the state level. Mississippi Governor Phil Bryant initially stayed out of the way, and HHS indicated it would work directly with Chaney. However, Bryant bowed under Tea Party pressure and threatened that his Medicaid agency would refuse to cooperate with the insurance department's exchange. The Obama administration reluctantly sided with Bryant, making Mississippi the only state to have an application for a state-based exchange rejected by the federal government (Jones 2017).

The need to fight on so many fronts was one important factor in the Obama administration's disastrous launch of HealthCare.gov on October 1, 2013, but many others contributed. This included the challenge of integrating databases from across multiple arms of government and a misguided reliance on Medicare.gov as a model for the website. But ultimately the site was launched successfully and became one of the centerpieces of the ACA. In the next section, we investigate the evidence of exchange success by looking beneath national statistics to unearth the importance of state participation.

The Record to Date

The goal of the exchanges was to improve coverage, access, affordability, and quality of benefits while maintaining sufficient commercial insurer competition to drive value. Initial enrollment in the exchanges was considerably lower than early estimates predicted due to technological glitches with HealthCare.gov and state-based exchange platforms, as well as the unaffordability of coverage options for higher-earning groups. The ACA had envisioned states taking the lead in advertising during open enrollment and so had not allocated much money to the federal government for this purpose. Former members of the Obama administration started Enroll America to go door to door and sign people up for coverage in large states that had rejected control of their exchange, such as Florida, North Carolina, and Texas. The Centers for Medicare and Medicaid Services had to take money from other ACA programs such as the Prevention Fund to pay for advertising.

Younger adults enrolled in coverage at lower rates than predicted, contributing to disappointing enrollment figures and risk pools that lacked healthier enrollees (Kliff 2014). By the end of 2013, politicians and pundits created a swirling sense that the exchanges were an impending disaster, with House Speaker John Boehner declaring he did not think the exchanges in particular and the ACA in general were "ever going to work" (Parkinson 2013).

Despite these dismal predictions, after a rocky start exchange enrollment increased and premiums were lower than predicted (Glied, Arora, and Solis-Roman 2015). Between 2013 and 2016, the portion of the total US population covered by nongroup private coverage grew from 3% to 7% (KFF 2017). This increase might seem modest, but one estimate suggests that nearly 40% of ACA-related coverage gains in 2014 were driven by the premium subsidies offered in the exchanges (Frean, Gruber, and Sommers 2016).

From 2016 to 2019, exchange enrollment slightly declined nationally. Considerable volatility in premiums arose as the Trump administration eliminated the cost-sharing reduction payments, slashed funding for enrollment assistance, and expanded access to ACA-noncompliant plans, and then Congress zeroed out the penalty for the individual mandate (KFF 2019). The exchanges have been remarkably resilient to these attacks due to strategic state responses and the enduring value of exchange coverage. For example, in response to the elimination of cost-sharing reduction payments, many states increased the price of their benchmark silver plan, a strategy known as "silver loading." Because federal premium tax credits are calculated using the price of the second-lowest silver-tier plan, this strategy recouped the lost federal cost-sharing reduction payments in the form of tax credit dollars and helped stabilize exchange markets.

Paradoxically, the elimination of the cost-sharing reduction payments has increased exchange enrollment and lowered premium costs for many low- to middle-income consumers (CBO 2018). In 2018, zero-premium coverage was available to over half of exchange enrollees (Branham and DeLeire 2019). In 2019, average premiums fell for the first time since the ACA was implemented, though prices have increased for higher-income consumers ineligible for federal subsidies (KFF 2019). More insurers entered the exchanges than exited in 2019, and nationwide, premiums are expected to decrease slightly in 2020 (Fehr, Cox, and Levitt 2018; Fehr et al. 2018; Scott 2019). The beneficial effects of silver loading may have weakened what could have been a series of fatal blows to the exchanges. Trump administration policies have put the exchanges to an important test: without a mandate and with cheaper, skimpier plans just a click away, do consumers abandon exchange coverage? The evidence suggests many have decided to stay.

Yet national statistics mask significant state-level heterogeneity. Despite the federal policies designed to regulate the cost and quality of insurance options sold through the exchanges, variations in implementation efforts drive stark differences in coverage, access, competition, and affordability by state. The Supreme Court in 2015 could have dramatically raised the stakes of state decisions had it concluded in *King v. Burwell* that tax credits were available only in states that ran their own exchange. Even so, one study found that premium subsidies were nearly twice as effective at increasing health insurance coverage rates in states that opted to establish their own exchange rather than use the federal exchange (Frean, Gruber, and Sommers 2016). Larger effects of premium tax credits in states with local exchanges reflect a host of state-level factors that enhance take-up of subsidized insurance. States that run their own exchanges benefit from greater customization and the opportunity to integrate enrollment infrastructure efforts across state programs. Under state or state-federal partnership exchange models, states conduct marketing, outreach, and consumer assistance and run their own online eligibility and enrollment platforms.

State-run outreach efforts have become critical to stabilizing exchanges in recent years as the Trump administration drastically cut funding for open enrollment advertising and consumer assistance programs. In 2017, nearly 800 counties in states with federally facilitated exchanges did not have any federally funded navigation services (Galewitz 2018). In contrast, states that have state-based exchanges were able to supplant federal funding with local funds. In California, healthy risk pools and an above-average insurance sign-up rate are due in part to the state's considerable expenditures on outreach (Corlette and Schwab 2018). State leaders elected in 2018 recognized the potential benefits of local exchange administration, as five additional states have indicated intent to transition part or all of their exchange infrastructure to the state level by 2020–22 (Schwab and Volk 2019).

Whether a state adopted Medicaid expansion is another important decision that effects the stability of exchanges, as expansion states were more likely than nonexpansion states to have more carriers participating in their markets, lower premiums, and healthier risk pools (Gabel et al. 2018; Han et al. 2015; Semanskee, Cox, and Levitt 2016; Sen and DeLiere 2016). This correlation may be due to Medicaid expansion offering an alternative source of coverage for individuals with greater health needs, which kept potentially higher-cost individuals out of state exchanges, Medicaid managed care organizations having more experience covering lower-income and higher-need populations, and less disruptive insurance coverage churn. State investment in Medicaid enrollment outreach also raised awareness of all insurance options, public and private.

Carrier participation also differs widely by region. In 2019, a third of rating regions had only one participating insurer, with the majority concentrated in southern, rural states with lower median incomes (Gabel et al. 2018). Markets with more competition offer enhanced consumer choice and lower premiums, which increases enrollment (Van Payrs 2018). However, insurers that have maintained financial viability in the exchanges have largely done so through selective contracting for lower rates with a narrow network of providers. Exchange plans with limited networks are a concern nationally, as limited provider options may impose barriers to timely access to care. Narrow networks are an even greater concern in rural regions where provider shortages already existed.

Despite the successes some states have experienced, exchanges have some shortcomings that impact all states. For example, affordability remains an issue nationally, with nearly half of exchange enrollees exposed to full cost sharing and nearly 90% of those in the exchanges enrolled in high-deductible health plans (Dolan 2016). Out-of-pocket prescription drug costs are double those of the average employee plan (Thorpe, Allen, and Joski 2015). Further, actuarial values represented by metallic tiers in qualified health plans are realized for only a small proportion of enrollees with enough health care spending for their insurer to pay their allocated portion of the costs. Because of this, most exchange enrollees pay for the majority of their care out of pocket (Polyakova, Hua, and Bundorf 2017). Again, states vary in their efforts to rein in premium costs, with 12 states establishing reinsurance programs through section 1332 state innovation waivers to encourage insurer participation, spur competition, and offer lower-priced plans to consumers.

While national- and state-level challenges exist, the exchanges still represent improvement relative to the unregulated, expensive, and inequitable insurance markets that existed before the ACA. The ACA was created to deal with high rates of uninsurance among low- to middle-income workers who were left out of private and public options, and the exchanges have created coverage where none existed. But was the political turmoil avoidable, or was it inherent in the federalism structure of the ACA? We explore these questions next.

Learning from the ACA and the Future of Federalism in Health Reform

The ACA was designed to foster near-universal insurance coverage, and its approach to that goal was to devise federal baselines above which states would operate. Federalism was a politically pragmatic choice that seemed necessary to gathering votes for the law's passage and a structural governance choice that is often a default approach in American health reform. Federalism also predictably results in variability. While variation can translate into policy successes or failures, variation in health policy often leads to inequitable policy across states and disparities across populations.

States were supposed to run the exchanges because states historically have regulated insurance. But, the ACA's implementation has been inconsistent with its statutory design. The political litmus test of resistance to the ACA, combined with opposition through litigation, has made it so the states that ordinarily prioritize their own sovereign lawmaking authority decided to reject federal policy, and federal power actually expanded within their borders through the federal exchange. The adaptive, negotiated, dynamic federalism that HHS and states engaged in to create something between the federal- and state-run exchanges was not the federalism of the ACA as enacted but developed organically as a response to implementation hurdles (Gluck and Huberfeld 2018). These negotiations have not reflected the Supreme Court's constitutional concern—that states could not fend for themselves—in striking down the Medicaid expansion as "coercive" in *NFIB v. Sebelius*. Rather, this dynamic federalism demonstrated states are adept at making demands and extracting compromises from HHS, learning from other states, negotiating, and finding a way to get a little more.

Our account of the exchange implementation dynamics illuminates that no federal health care takeover has occurred. Indeed, the unevenness of state exchange implementation may indicate that the federal law of the ACA does not go far enough in creating a strong national baseline, precisely because this variability has weakened the policy goal of universal coverage. Varying levels of success across states reflect the design of the federal law. But states' successes and failures also reflect the negotiations that occurred to implement the ACA, which included state policy decisions to support or thwart the ACA at every stage. Notably, HHS Secretary Kathleen Sebelius and other officials in the Obama administration accepted state participation in many forms, regardless of the ACA's statutory design, so that hybrid and partnership exchanges also developed. These were not specifically contemplated by the ACA but arose in response to the political resistance to the law that was itself undermined by state insurance commissioners' and health care stakeholders' desire to see the law implemented. Perhaps most surprising, the vast majority of states have a hand in running the exchange in their own markets, whether or not they established any kind of state-based, partnership, hybrid, or other exchange.

So whether the ACA's new exchanges were successful very much depends on where one looks, as states both implemented and undercut the ACA during the Obama administration. Some states that tried to create their own exchanges failed, while other states that appeared hostile on the surface actually worked with the Obama administration behind the scenes. For example, both Oregon and Florida rely on the federal exchange platform, but their politics and policy desires have been very different, with

Oregon reliably counting as "blue" (tried to create an exchange but failed) and Florida counting as "red" (never created its own exchange). In other words, the federalism story is much more complex than the standard account that two-thirds of states did not implement state-based exchanges. The fact of a state relying on the federal exchange does not begin to tell us everything about that state's engagement with the ACA or whether or why that state experienced significant increases in coverage.

Further, resisting creation of a state-run exchange was just one way that states undermined the ACA during the Obama administration. For example, we noted above that the interplay between exchanges and Medicaid expansion has been important. While nearly half of the individuals who are uninsured could enroll through an exchange with federal tax subsidies, these remaining uninsured are living in Medicaid nonexpansion states— states that have resisted ACA implementation in all of its federalism dimensions. These ACA-hostile states have higher rates of uninsurance and poorer performance on the other metrics of health policy success. Yet, paradoxically, some states also worked with HHS to expand Medicaid and implement exchanges with state-specific names and special rules attuned to the politics of the state—though these were acts of state resistance to Obamacare (similar to Governor Brownback's vision described above), ultimately such engagement helped facilitate the exchanges' success.

The Trump administration made no secret of its hostility to the law; President Trump's first executive order was a directive to limit the regulatory scope of the ACA. The administration took steps to thwart the ACA's goal of universal coverage, such as cutting navigator funding, decreasing advertising for open enrollment, limiting the open enrollment period, and destabilizing the small markets of the exchanges by allowing short-term plans to be sold as ACA compliant. The administration has been undermining exchange enrollment while at the same time allowing states to create barriers to Medicaid expansion enrollment for the people newly eligible under the ACA, such as work requirements—again, the fate of the exchanges and Medicaid expansion have been intertwined.

Despite the challenging road to implementation and multiple legislative attacks, the exchanges have become a standard building block of the American health insurance architecture. In fact, the Republican replacement bills, such as the American Health Care Act of 2017, included the same basic framework of an exchange with consumer protections and premium tax credits. The House Republican bill did include important changes at the margins, such as increasing the rating band to 5:1 and tying premiums to age instead of income, but these were not supported by Senate Republicans. And, these were not legally or structurally significant changes relative to what the ACA already created—a federalism-dependent, highly regulated, publicly supported insurance market.

Yet, the role of federalism in the success or failure of the exchanges is ultimately hard to measure, in part because states' policy choices have cut both ways. Some states undercut the law during the early years, leading to challenges to the law, such as *NFIB v. Sebelius* and *King v. Burwell*. States also limited the reach of the federal exchange by enacting nullification laws, which were of no legal consequence but contributed to public confusion about the ACA's existence. And states' refusal to engage with HHS publicly also undermined accountability for the exchange implementation, which made it harder for voters to know who was responsible for the law's successes and failures.

For all of this confusion and resistance, the nation's uninsurance rate at the end of the Obama administration was the lowest it had ever been, at 8.6% by some measures. While the exchanges do not cover a large percentage of the population, they provide subsidized access to insurance markets for those who have been stuck outside of both public and private insurance, playing a key role in expanding coverage for low-income and part-time workers.

Conclusion

The fight over health insurance exchanges over the last 10 years is a fascinating case study in what happens when preferences over policy and federalism conflict with partisan goals. Exchanges were initially a bipartisan idea that became ideologically charged only as they became wrapped in the broader party politics of Obamacare. After congressional Republicans failed to block the ACA's passage, some of their state-level counterparts used their role in implementing the exchanges to attempt postenactment obstructionism that they hoped would unravel the entire law, even if it meant forgoing funding and ceding control to the federal government. Perhaps this was a risk they were willing to take, given that they did not truly oppose the idea of an exchange.

Our account demonstrates that the states that have engaged with the ACA most consistently appear to have experienced greater exchange-related success. But each aspect of states' engagement with or resistance to the ACA must be counted to fully paint this picture, with significant variation between states. This variation should give pause to those considering next steps in health reform, because state variation can mean innovation and improvement but also lack of coverage, disparities, and diminished access to care.

The 2020 presidential election approaches as we contemplate the ACA's signing anniversary. Throughout the primary debates, a core group of Democratic contenders have advocated for an incremental health reform approach that builds on the exchanges, not just by expanding the exchanges' tax subsidies but also by building the public option so quickly discarded in 2009. Some have advocated for dismantling the private provision of health insurance altogether. President Trump has said he will have a new health reform proposal in January 2021, with no further detail, but if 2017 is a guide, a new proposal is unlikely to include a dismantling of the exchanges. In fact, the Trump administration has tried to use the messiness of federalism and the fight over exchanges to both blame-shift and credit-claim, that is, taking credit for any positive developments—such as decreases in premiums—and blaming President Obama, congressional Democrats, and state leaders for any struggles.

Regardless of how new health reform proposals play out, a certain portion of health care decision making is nearly guaranteed to be punted to the states. (Even Senator Bernie Sanders's Medicare for All bill keeps the Medicaid program for long-term care coverage.) As we've learned from the ACA's exchanges, state-level cooperation and opposition are likely to play a major role in shaping the success or failure of future health reform.

▪ ▪ ▪

David K. Jones is associate professor at the Boston University School of Public Health. He is the author of *Exchange Politics: Opposing Obamacare in Battleground States* (2017). His work has appeared in the *New York Times*, the *Washington Post*, and the *Wall Street Journal*, among others. He has been awarded the Academy-Health Outstanding Dissertation Award and the John D. Thompson Prize for Young Investigators by the Association of University Programs in Health Administration. dkjones@bu.edu

Sarah H. Gordon is assistant professor in the Department of Health Law, Policy, and Management at the Boston University School of Public Health. She is a quantitative researcher studying the effects of state policies on insurance coverage and health care utilization. In her prior work, she examined disenrollment from Affordable Care Act Marketplaces and compared the effects of public coverage versus subsidized private coverage on costs, quality, and utilization of care. Her broad interests are in state health policy, access to care, and health equity.

Nicole Huberfeld is professor of health law, ethics, and human rights and professor of law at Boston University. Her scholarship explores the cross section of health law and constitutional law, often addressing health reform (especially Medicaid), federalism, and the spending power. She is author of two health law casebooks and many book chapters and articles, including "What Is Federalism in Healthcare For?" (*Stanford Law Review*, 2018, with Abbe Gluck), a 5-year study of the federalism dynamics of the implementation of the ACA, and "Federalizing Medicaid" (2011), cited in the first Supreme Court decision on the ACA.

References

Branham, Douglas Keith, and Thomas DeLeire. 2019. "Zero-Premium Health Insurance Plans Became More Prevalent in Federal Marketplaces in 2018." *Health Affairs* 38, no. 5: 820–25.

CBO (Congressional Budget Office). 2018. "Federal Subsidies for Health Insurance Coverage for People under Age 65: 2018–2028." May. www.cbo.gov/system/files /2018-06/53826-healthinsurancecoverage.pdf.

Corlette, Sabrina, and Rachel Schwab. 2018. "States Lean In as the Federal Government Cuts Back on Navigator and Advertising Funding for the ACA's Sixth Open Enrollment." Commonwealth Fund, October 26. www.commonwealthfund.org /blog/2018/states-lean-federal-government-cuts-back-navigator-and-advertising -funding.

Dolan, Rachel. 2016. "High-Deductible Health Plans." *Health Affairs*, February 4. www-healthaffairs-org.revproxy.brown.edu/do/10.1377/hpb20160204.950878/full/.

Fehr, Rachel, Cynthia Cox, and Larry Levitt. 2019. "Insurer Participation on ACA Marketplaces, 2014–2020." Kaiser Family Foundation, November 21. www.kff.org /health-reform/issue-brief/insurer-participation-on-aca-marketplaces-2014-2020/.

Fehr, Rachel, Rabah Kamal, and Cynthia Cox. 2018. "How ACA Marketplace Premiums Are Changing by County in 2020." Kaiser Family Foundation, November 7. www.kff.org/health-costs/issue-brief/how-aca-marketplace-premium sare-changing-by-county-in-2019.

Frean, Molly, Jonathan Gruber, and Benjamin D. Sommers. 2016. "Disentangling the ACA's Coverage Effects—Lessons for Policymakers." *New England Journal of Medicine* 375: 1605–08.

Gabel, Jon R., Heidi Whitmore, Sam Stromberg, and Matthew Green. 2018. "Why Are the Health Insurance Marketplaces Thriving in Some States but Struggling in Others?" Commonwealth Fund, November 15. www.commonwealthfund.org /publications/issue-briefs/2018/nov/marketplaces-thriving-some-states-struggling -others.

Galewitz, Phil. 2018. "Short on Federal Funding, Obamacare Enrollment Navigators Switch Tactics." *Kaiser Health News*, November 30. khn.org/news/short-on -federal-funding-obamacare-enrollment-navigators-switch-tactics/.

Glied, Sherry, Anupama Arora, and Claudia Solis-Roman. 2015. "The CBO's Crystal Ball: How Well Did It Forecast the Effects of the Affordable Care Act?" Commonwealth Fund, December 15. www.commonwealthfund.org/publications/issue-briefs/2015/dec/cbos-crystal-ball-how-well-did-it-forecast-effects-affordable.

Gluck, Abbe R., and Nicole Huberfeld. 2018. "What Is Federalism in Healthcare For?" *Stanford Law Review* 70, no. 6: 1689.

Haislmaier, Edmund. 2006. "The Significance of Massachusetts Health Reform." Heritage Foundation, April 11. www.heritage.org/research/reports/2006/04/the-significance-of-massachusetts-health-reform.

Han, Xuesong, Binh T. Nguyen, Jeffrey Drope, and Ahmedin Jemal. 2015. "Health-Related Outcomes among the Poor: Medicaid Expansion vs. Non-expansion States." *PLoS One* 10, no. 12: e0144429.

Jones, David K. 2017. *Exchange Politics*. Oxford University Press: New York.

Jones, David K., Katharine W. V. Bradley, and Jonathan Oberlander. 2014. "Pascal's Wager: Health Insurance Exchanges, Obamacare, and the Republican Dilemma." *Journal of Health Politics, Policy and Law* 39, no. 1: 97–137.

Jost, Timothy S. 2010. "Implementation and Enforcement of Health Care Reform—Federal versus State Government." *New England Journal of Medicine* 362: e2. doi: 10.1056/NEJMp0911636.

KFF (Kaiser Family Foundation). 2010. "Kaiser Health Tracking Poll." June. www.kff.org/wp-content/uploads/2013/01/8082-f.pdf.

KFF (Kaiser Family Foundation). 2017. "Health Insurance Coverage of the Total Population." www.kff.org/other/state-indicator/total-population/?currentTimeframe=0&sortModel=%7B%22colId%22:%22Location%22,%22sort%22:%22asc%22%7D (accessed February 7, 2020).

KFF (Kaiser Family Foundation). 2019. "Marketplace Effectuated Enrollment and Financial Assistance." www.kff.org/other/state-indicator/effectuated-marketplace-enrollment-and-financial-assistance/?currentTimeframe=0&sortModel=%7B%22colId%22:%22Location%22,%22sort%22:%22asc%22%7D (accessed November 25, 2019).

Kliff, Sarah. 2014. "One in Four Obamacare Enrollees Are Young Adults. That's Below the Target." *Vox*, January 13. www.washingtonpost.com/news/wonk/wp/2014/01/13/one-in-four-obamacare-enrollees-are-young-adults-thats-below-the-target/.

Mooney, Kevin. 2011. "ObamaCare Opponents Differ Sharply over Strategy at ALEC Conference." *Pelican Post*, August 8.

Morton, Heather. 2013. "Insurance State Regulators—Selection and Term Statutes." National Conference of State Legislatures, April 12. www.ncsl.org/research/financial-services-and-commerce/insurance-state-regulators-selection-and-term-stat.aspx.

Parkinson, John. 2013. "Boehner Predicts Obamacare Will 'Never Work.'" ABC News, November 13. www.abcnews.go.com/blogs/politics/2013/11/boehner-predicts-obamacare-will-never-work/.

Polyakova, Maria, Lynn Mei Hua, and M. Kate Bundorf. 2017. "Marketplace Plans Provide Risk Protection, but Actuarial Values Overstate Realized Coverage for Most Enrollees." *Health Affairs* 36, no. 12: 2078–84.

Schwab, Rachel, and JoAnn Volk. 2019. "States Looking to Run Their Own Health Insurance Marketplace See Opportunity for Funding, Flexibility." Commonwealth Fund, June 28. www.commonwealthfund.org/blog/2019/states-looking-to-run-their -own-health-insurance-marketplace-see-opportunity.

Scott, Dylan. 2019. "2020 Obamacare Premiums Are on Track for Smallest Increases Ever." *Vox*, October 28. www.vox.com/policy-and-politics/2019/10/28/20936573 /obamacare-health-insurance-open-enrollment-2020.

Semanskee, Ashley, Cynthia Cox, and Larry Levitt. 2016. "Data Note: Effect of State Decisions on State Risk Pools." Kaiser Family Foundation, October. files.kff.org /attachment/Data-Note-Effect-of-State-Decisions-on-State-Risk-Pools.

Sen, Aditi P., and Thomas DeLeire. 2016. "The Effect of Medicaid Expansion on Marketplace Premiums." Department of Health and Human Services, ASPE Issue Brief, September 6. aspe.hhs.gov/system/files/pdf/206761/McaidExpMktplPrem .pdf.

Thorpe, Kenneth E., Lindsay Allen, and Peter Joski. 2015. "Out-of-Pocket Prescription Costs under a Typical Silver Plan Are Twice as High as They Are in the Average Employer Plan." *Health Affairs* 34, no. 10: 1695–1703.

Van Payrs, Jessica. 2018. "ACA Marketplace Premiums Grew More Rapidly in Areas with Monopoly Insurers than in Areas with More Competition." *Health Affairs* 37, no. 8: 1243–51.

What Is the Affordable Care Act a Case of? Understanding the ACA through the Comparative Method

Holly Jarman
Scott L. Greer
University of Michigan

Abstract International comparisons of US health care are common but mostly focus on comparing its performance to peers or asking why the United States remains so far from universal coverage. Here the authors ask how other comparative research could shed light on the unusual politics and structure of US health care and how the US experience could bring more to international conversations about health care and the welfare state. After introducing the concept of casing—asking what the Affordable Care Act (ACA) might be a case of—the authors discuss different "casings" of the ACA: complex legislation, path dependency, demos-constraining institutions, deep social cleavages, segmentalism, or the persistence of the welfare state. Each of these pictures of the ACA has strong support in the US-focused literature. Each also cases the ACA as part of a different experience shared with other countries, with different implications for how to analyze it and what we can learn from it. The final section discusses the implications for selecting cases that might shed light on the US experience and that make the United States look less exceptional and more tractable as an object of research.

Keywords ACA, comparative politics, health care reform

During debates on the Affordable Care Act (ACA), reforms in the legislation were frequently compared to health systems in other countries. On the pro-reform side, comparative data from health systems around the world were used in political debate to demonstrate how comparatively expensive yet mediocre US health care had become and to argue the case for reform (Peterson 2011). Among the ACA's opponents, images of "socialist" or authoritarian health care systems were used to invoke fear

Journal of Health Politics, Policy and Law, Vol. 45, No. 4, August 2020
DOI 10.1215/03616878-8255589 © 2020 by Duke University Press

about the ACA and what it would mean for the future role of the federal government (Ehlke 2011). Commentators continued to talk about Canadian-, Singaporean-, French-, or Dutch-style health care or "single payer" or "universal health care," without much context or analysis (Brown 2012; Marmor, Freeman, and Okma 2005). This tendency lives on in discussions about the ACA and ideas like "Medicare for all." Phrases like *single payer* are still incorrectly used by the Left as shorthand for "good health care system" (Greer, Jarman, and Donnelly 2019; Sparer, Brown, and Jacobs, 2009).

It might be a good time, therefore, to revisit the question of how best to compare the US health care system to those in other countries. Ten years after the passage of the ACA, how should we make sense of the reforms from a comparative perspective? Can we make such comparisons truly meaningful when the United States seems to be, at least superficially, an "exceptional case"?

Understanding something as complex as the ACA, or US health care policy, in a comparative context is a significant endeavor that few have undertaken (Marmor and Klein 2012; Tuohy 1999, 2018; White 2013). But we can apply some thinking from comparative social inquiry to make the process easier. The following sections draw from literature on the comparative method in order to think about how we might define the ACA as a phenomenon and how we might compare it to other cases. A vast, cross-disciplinary body of literature in the social sciences examines different ways to define, select, and compare cases. Although this body of work is far too voluminous to examine extensively here, we provide some useful starting points for generating comparative insights that can help us to understand the ACA in a new light.

Casing as an Act of Research

One of the first things that comparative scholars will often do when working on a project is to try to construct a "case" by figuring out the boundaries of the phenomenon to be studied. Ragin (1992) describes the process of constructing a case, or "casing," as a fundamental act of research. Researchers move back and forth between considering their case in the light of relevant theoretical ideas and empirical evidence in a process known as retroduction (Ragin 2011). This is far closer to the actual practice of research than much of the standard discussion of inductive and deductive research. In reality, most findings are not driven by the testing of a prior induction or the atheoretical induction of facts. They come from researchers who realize what is truly interesting about their topic as they move more deeply into both relevant theory and their case. Casing permits what we most want: the identification of portable causal arguments that can be convincingly used in some cases, as well as the scope of conditions under which they cannot be used (Falleti and Lynch 2009). When investigating complex social phenomena, the process of casing will almost certainly continue throughout the study, with researchers refining the boundaries of what their case is as their understanding grows.

With these insights in mind, how should we begin to "case" the ACA? After a decade of complex implementation, the ACA is much more than the law itself or the surrounding political debate. Put more specifically, what is the ACA a case of? What kinds of theory illuminate it, and what kinds of theory does it build? In the context of current debates in comparative politics, some promising ways to case the ACA include defining it as complex legislation, path dependency, demos-constraining institutions, deep social cleavages, segmentalism, persistence of the welfare state, or mandatory private insurance. These case definitions are by no means exhaustive. In a real study, researchers would change their conceptual understanding of the case throughout the project through the process of gathering and synthesizing information. Nevertheless, running through some examples is perhaps the best way to show how casing the ACA might work in practice. Each of these different casings highlights a dimension of US health care politics with international equivalents.

Uniquely Complex Legislation

For example, is the ACA a case of an American style of uniquely complex legislation? An increasing number of scholars have written about how public policy in the United States (especially health policy) is needlessly complex and builds in layers of interests at the expense of accountability, traceability, effectiveness, or efficiency. Whether we call it the delegated welfare state (Morgan and Campbell 2011), the submerged welfare state (Mettler 2011), the hidden welfare state (Howard 1999), or kludgeocracy (Teles 2012), the complexity of US social policy and its pernicious effects are a focus of much scholarship today (Greer 2018). The ACA is certainly a case of a very complex and indirect piece of legislation. Even politically and administratively simpler coverage mechanisms, such as extension of state insurance regulation, were complex and largely disguised from voters who might give politicians credit (Béland, Rocco, and Waddan 2016).

This intuition and extensive exploration of policy dynamics in the United States have not, however, been matched with efforts to see if US policy is indeed such an outlier in complexity, and why. US policy making is more elaborate than that of the Westminster systems, such as those in the United Kingdom or Canada. But are US policy processes really more complex and riddled with rent seekers than public policy making in France, or more obscure and ineffective than public policy processes in Italy? For that matter, is the relative simplicity of Westminster policymaking matched by relatively simpler policies?

One reason these authors give for the complexity of public policy is the fragmentation of the US political system, combined with its enormously dense interest group infrastructure, which means that interest groups can defend themselves against efforts to rationalize the system or effectively contain costs. Much of the complexity of the ACA comes from Democrats' decision to sidestep conflict by leaving most of the previous system in place (Oberlander 2016), which helped secure passage and make implementation possible at the price of extending the complexity of health policy. In a variant of this argument, Drutman (2015) persuasively argues that lobbyists, eager to demonstrate their return on investment, might also be making all policy more complex than it needs to be. This might help explain the lobby-filled US health care world, but it might also explain EU policy making, where legislation is just as complex, with just as many lobbyists eager to demonstrate the need for lobbying.

Path Dependency

Most of the authors in the literature on complex public policy point to interest group activity as a key driver of the complexity they identify. But if the ACA, and US politics and public policy in general, are more complex than other countries with more waste, then maybe it is too simple to blame only interest groups. A powerful explanation for the complexity and partiality of US coverage politics can be found in path dependency, a concept with a particularly strong lineage in comparative politics research. The case is perhaps best put in the case of US health policy by Mayes (2004). Path dependency arguments emphasize the extent to which decisions at one time lock in costs and benefits and trigger positive- and negative-sum dynamics. Even if another approach would be better, the costs of transitioning to it are now so big that it is impossible, and we need not look to further explanations such as partisanship or interest groups in understanding why. In other words, once you have taken the wrong turn, turning around and going back hours later is so costly that you don't. Thus, for example, one might argue that once Medicare or employer-sponsored health care were established in policy, they created their own constituencies among elites and the public, became harder to reform, and jointly became an obstacle to a coverage reform. The evidence for such a thesis is not hard to find (e.g., Campbell 2003; Gottschalk 1999; Klein 2003; Mettler and Soss 2004; Oberlander 2003; Quadagno 2005; Tuohy 1999).

Path dependency arguments are powerful in explaining that divergence sometimes just *is*. At the same time, path dependency arguments also have some weaknesses that comparative politics scholars have been trying to address (Mahoney and Thelen 2015). First, while they produce an interesting search for critical junctures in history, they do less explanatory work now—each country ends up on its own path. Second, this search for critical junctures can turn into a swamp (Brown 2010): At what point, exactly, did the United States embark irrevocably on the path leading to today? Was any particular trajectory a necessary result of a given event? Third, there is no guarantee that any given policy triggers a self-reinforcing feedback loop (Oberlander and Weaver 2015). Those opposed to the policy and its effects might be able to mobilize against it and make countervailing policies that just lead to stalemate or to policy cycling (Tuohy 2018).

Demos-Constraining Institutions

If the ACA is more, or differently, kludgeocratic, delegated, and submerged than the policy of other countries—it is certainly less universal—and if the difference is not just due to history, then is the outcome because of the number and strength of demos-constraining institutions, which explicitly constrain democracy, in the US political system (Stepan and Linz 2011)? Demos-constraining institutions can work in two ways. One is through federal-level veto points (e.g., the Supreme Court, the independence of two legislative branches and the executive, or the filibuster). The other is through fragmentation (e.g., dividing the people into multiple jurisdictions, such as 50 states and about 90,000 local governments), which promotes intergovernmental competition and raises the costs of enacting policy by demanding enactment in more jurisdictions. Medicaid expansion in the ACA showed them working together: one veto player, the Supreme Court, rewrote the law to make expansion optional for states, which created 50 new venues in which to contest the policy. American demos-constraining institutions are both strikingly numerous by international standards and, in many cases, particularly strong, as with the absurdly malapportioned

Senate, its filibuster, or the Electoral College (Stepan and Linz 2011). It thus should be no surprise that the United States has such a problem of political, social, and economic inequality: its institutions impede the most effective action against such problems (Stepan and Linz 2011).

The United States is certainly poor at delivering policy outcomes that reflect the overall preferences of its population. Page and Gilens (2017) contentiously argued that there was no relationship between the percentage of the American public who support a policy and its likelihood of passage. There is no clear comparative literature that tells us whether the United States is more or less responsive than other countries. The ACA in this perspective, though, is not particularly ambitious legislation compared to universal health care, but it is something like the best that could be got through American political institutions as they currently stand (Tuohy 2018). This account is highly plausible and fits with studies of other complex and demos-constraining political environments, such as Brazil (Arretche 2013; Segatto and Béland 2019) and the European Union (Héritier 1999; Obinger, Leibfried, and Castles 2005). In those polities, any kind of policy success depends on creativity and clever bypasses of demos-constraining institutions—a phenomenon that Americanists recognize as "unorthodox lawmaking" (Sinclair 2016).

Deeper Social Cleavages

Of course, these demos-constraining institutions, from the beginning, have been sustained by those who do not benefit from more democracy, including slaveholders and the beneficiaries of Jim Crow, as well as other interests that would not benefit from the passage of popular redistributive policies. So perhaps both the institutions and the policies reflect deeper social cleavages, notably those of race and perhaps also of class. This perspective flips the preceding one, as when Riker (1964: 155) said of state's rights that "if one disapproves of racism, one should disapprove of federalism." If American institutions developed as a long series of compromises with antidemocratic or undemocratic forces that are still at work today, should we instead focus on those forces and view institutions as endogenous to that explanation?

Marx (1998), for example, shed considerable light on the United States by comparing it to two other countries with similar legacies of white supremacy: Brazil and South Africa. Lieberman (2009) likewise demonstrated the negative effects of racial hierarchies and politics on AIDS policies with an argument that could well apply to the US. There certainly is persuasive evidence that the ACA was "racialized" in the eyes of many whites (Grogan and Park 2017; Tesler 2011) and that this is part of a larger rise of white identity and nationalism (Maxwell and Shields 2019; Morone 2018). From this perspective, the United States is in a catch-22: racism that manifests in inherited institutions, in public opinion, and in organized political forces impedes redistribution even when it would be in most whites' interests, but at the same time it is a redistributive welfare state that enables progress toward racial equity (Katznelson 2005; Lieberman 1998).

Through that lens, the ACA, while it extends coverage and promotes equity in a variety of ways (Grogan 2017), is still only a partial coverage extension by the standards of other rich countries, and it came with a furious and racialized backlash. Perhaps it could be read as just another episode in intertwined battles over race and redistribution, or another case of the extension of universal social programs that follows on a democratic advance. The backlash against the ACA, which cost Democrats congressional seats in 2010 (Nyhan et al. 2012; Saldin 2011), could in this casing be read as another one of the backlashes that follow on civil rights victories. Pursuing the implications of all the work identifying race as a key variable in America health politics drives the casing process, and comparisons, in new comparative directions—toward the other societies marked by industrial chattel slavery and racial hierarchy, which are found principally in the New World, rather than long established states in a European continent marked by centuries of state and nationalist efforts to create homogeneity. It equally, though, raises complex questions of causality, since institutions are not perfect reflections of today's politics, and in public opinion beliefs about race work through complex ideas of "deservingness" (Lynch and Gollust 2010).

Segmentalism

Another, related way to view the extension of health care access in the United States is as part of a push, led by the Left, to reduce segmentalism (sometimes also known as stratification) in health care policy. In this case, Latin American or some East Asian countries, rather than European ones, might be the most useful comparators (Haggard and Kaufman 2008). Latin America and southern Europe have histories of "segmentalist" systems in which particular groups have different health care access, with some groups, such as the workers of the most favored companies, enjoying good benefits and some others frozen out entirely or dependent on a thin public safety net (Martínez Franzoni and Sánchez-Ancochea 2018). By such a definition, the United States is, like Chile, Brazil, or Mexico, a country whose politics are shaped by a segmentalist legacy and where the debate is about whether and how to universalize its health services (Greer, Jarman, and Donnelly 2019; Greer and Méndez 2015).

Persistence of the Welfare State

But despite being flawed and hard to claim credit for, and being caught in a backlash of tremendous force, the ACA persists. Is the ACA best viewed as a case of the persistence of the welfare state? Since the 1980s, scholars of comparative welfare states found not so much a rollback as a slowing of the extension of the welfare state in what is known as the "new politics" of welfare (Pierson 1996). The basic logic is that in any system it is hard to take away benefits that people currently enjoy (Brooks and Manza 2007). Veto points in the institutions will make it harder to shrink the welfare by empowering both interests that oppose cuts and interests that block change or extension. If the program does lose its effectiveness, it probably will not be through big legislative changes. Rather, it will suffer "policy drift," in which failure to update a policy means that over time it ceases to fulfill, and perhaps even undermines, its original goals (Hacker 2004). Of course, the argument that politicians will avoid overt retrenchment is a poor fit with the actual experience of the ACA, which *was* almost repealed despite obvious political and policy reasons not to (Hacker and Pierson 2018). America's numerous veto points just barely saved the ACA, but from a partisan assault whose magnitude most theorists of new politics would hardly have expected.

Comparing the ACA to Other Cases

The next step in applying the comparative method is to select further cases for comparison. Once researchers have at least some preliminary under-standing of what the ACA is a case of, they can begin to think about it not just as a case in isolation but as part of a constellation of cases that can be grouped into sets or categorized in different ways. In other words, how does the ACA, as a case of X, relate to other cases of X? What dimensions of the US experience allow us to create meaningful comparisons that contribute to our international as well as US expertise?

Again, selecting cases is an act of research. Case selection is a preoc-cupation of literature in comparative politics because it is central to the credibility of the findings, shapes the kinds of lessons that might be learned, and above all, determines the scope conditions for any generalization. Done badly, comparative analysis can degenerate into simple impres-sionistic analogy. Efforts to develop an approach to case selection based on frequentist statistical methods (King, Keohane, and Verba 1994) also tend to fail (Brady and Collier 2010) because treating qualitative comparison simply as a way to address "small *n* problems" does not exploit the richness of a case as a set of interacting variables. More productive efforts to develop case selection have focused on just that richness: identifying subtler ways that variables interact within cases over time in order to tease out configurations of variables and their effects.

Attention to case selection equally allows us to identify less valid inferences. For example, there are probably too many UK-US comparisons, since a shared language and an English tendency to borrow fashionable American phrases like *population health* and *accountable care organizations* can distract from the fact that in important respects they are very different polities. The highly centralized, executive-focused United Kingdom, the size of the public National Health Service systems, and the strong concept of positive social citizenship among UK citizens all make it more of a contrast than a suitable comparison with the United States. It is highly unlikely, for example, that endless debates about putative "Americanization" of the British health system have brought much clarity to UK policy conversations (Powell, Béland, and Waddan 2018).

Each of the six "casings" of the ACA we identify above points to a different set of comparisons that would shed light on the US experience and future, while contributing to an international conversation. If the question is just how distinctively complex US legislation is and why, then cases from the Netherlands, Switzerland, and Italy can teach us about the politics of complexity. If the question is about how path dependency works, then identifying similar cases at key junctures can be illuminating, for example, Canada in the 1970s (Maioni 1998). If the question is how demos-constraining institutions shape the United States and how they may be worked around, then the veto-ridden European Union is a case, as well as other wealthy states such as Switzerland, where policy making is built around anticipation and management of vetoes. If the question is how to understand deep social cleavages, particularly the changing racial politics of health in divided societies, then a more delicate operation is needed to seek lessons from quite distant countries, such as Brazil or South Africa, where racial inequalities and politics are important to any distributive question. If the question is how to understand segmentalist legacies, adding an international dimension to the extensive literature on path-dependent and interest-group-reinforced segmentalism in the United States, then relevant cases would be countries that substantially overcame segmentalism (e.g., Spain and Brazil; Linos 2013) and ones that failed to do so, as well as the hybrids that have evolved (Wong 2004).

Once we "case" the ACA, then we can see it in a new light and see what lessons can be exchanged with the rest of the world. It might not be comfortable to compare the United States to Brazil or South Africa, or an easy research project to figure out Japanese health care financing and politics in order to shed light on the experience of others (Schoppa 2006; White 2013), but those projects can be revealing if done with rigorous attention to case selection and inference.

Conclusion

Comparisons of the US health system are often made with an overt agenda, typically of showing its extraordinary expense, inequity, and mediocre results (Cohn 2009; Reid 2010; Schneider et al. 2017). While understanding these differences may be important, viewing the United States as an exceptional case, or just a poor performer, constrains our thinking about both health problems and potential solutions.

To the extent that the United States is a case of a system with too many veto players, we can expect partial and fragmentary legislation, but equally, the experiences of other countries show that complexity and indirection of the ACA and much US policy might not be inevitable. The United States stands out relative to European countries for the depth and historical importance of its domestic racial cleavage and its segmentalism, but those phenomena are also ones that many Latin American and southern European countries face and are addressing in their politics. In other words, if the United States is cased carefully, there is scope to introduce new thinking about the ACA and the rest of the world into our health policy research.

■ ■ ■

Holly Jarman is the John G. Searle Assistant Professor of Health Management and Policy at the University of Michigan. As a political scientist, she examines the impact of economic regulations on domestic health policies in Europe, Canada, and the United States. She has published more than 30 peer-reviewed articles in such journals as the *American Journal of Public Health, Milbank Quarterly, Lancet, BMJ Tobacco Control*, and *European Journal of Public Health*. Her books include *Everything You Always Wanted to Know about European Union Health Policies But Were Afraid to Ask* (2019) and *The Politics of Trade and Tobacco Control* (2015). hjarman@umich.edu

Scott L. Greer is professor of health management and policy, global public health, and political science at the University of Michigan School of Public Health. He researches the politics of health policies, with a special focus on the impact of federalism on health care. His recent books include *Everything You Always Wanted to Know about European Union Health Policies but Were Afraid to Ask* (2019) and *Federalism and Social Policy: Patterns of Redistribution in Eleven Democracies* (2019).

References

Arretche, Marta. 2013. "Constraining or Demos-Enabling Federalism? Political Institutions and Policy Change in Brazil." *Journal of Politics in Latin America* 5, no. 2: 133–50.

Béland, Daniel, Philip Rocco, and Alex Waddan. 2016. *Obamacare Wars: Federalism, State Politics, and the Affordable Care Act*. Lawrence: University Press of Kansas.

Brady, Henry E., and David Collier. 2010. *Rethinking Social Inquiry: Diverse Tools, Shared Standards*. Lanham, MD: Rowman and Littlefield.

Brooks, Clem, and Jeff Manza. 2007. *Why Welfare States Persist: The Importance of Public Opinion in Democracies*. Chicago: University of Chicago Press.

Brown, Lawrence D. 2010. "Pedestrian Paths: Why Path-Dependence Theory Leaves Health Policy Analysis Lost in Space." *Journal of Health Politics, Policy and Law* 35, no. 4: 643–61.

Brown, Lawrence D. 2012. "The Fox and the Grapes: Is Real Reform Beyond Reach in the United States?" *Journal of Health Politics, Policy and Law* 37, no. 4: 587–609.

Campbell, Andrea Louise. 2003. *How Policies Make Citizens: Senior Political Activism and the American Welfare State*. Princeton, NJ: Princeton University Press.

Cohn, Jonathan. 2009. *Sick: The True Story of America's Health Care Crisis—and the People Who Pay the Price*. New York: HarperCollins.

Drutman, Lee. 2015. *The Business of America Is Lobbying: How Corporations Became Politicized and Politics Became More Corporate*. New York: Oxford University Press.

Ehlke, Daniel. 2011. "The Political Abuse of International Health System Comparisons." *Journal of Health Services Research and Policy* 16, no. 3: 197–89.

Falleti, Tulia G., and Julia F. Lynch. 2009. "Context and Causal Mechanisms in Political Analysis." *Comparative Political Studies* 42, no. 9: 1143–66.

Gottschalk, Marie. 1999. "The Elusive Goal of Universal Health Care in the US: Organized Labor and the Institutional Straitjacket of the Private Welfare State." *Journal of Policy History* 11, no. 4: 367–98.

Greer, Scott L. 2018. "The Politics of Bad Policy in the United States." *Perspectives on Politics* 16, no. 2: 455–59.

Greer, Scott L., Holly Jarman, and Peter D. Donnelly. 2019. "Lessons for the United States from Single-Payer Systems." *American Journal of Public Health* 109, no. 11: 1493–96.

Greer, Scott L., and Claudio A. Méndez. 2015. "Universal Health Coverage: A Political Struggle and Governance Challenge." *American Journal of Public Health* 105, suppl. 5: S637–39.

Grogan, Colleen M. 2017. "How the ACA Addressed Health Equity and What Repeal Would Mean." *Journal of Health Politics, Policy and Law* 42, no. 5: 985–93.

Grogan, Colleen M., and Sunggeun Park. 2017. "The Racial Divide in State Medicaid Expansions." *Journal of Health Politics, Policy and Law* 42, no. 3: 539–72.

Hacker, Jacob S. 2004. "Privatizing Risk without Privatizing the Welfare State: The Hidden Politics of Social Policy Retrenchment in the United States." *American Political Science Review* 98, no. 2: 243–260.

Hacker, Jacob S., and Paul Pierson. 2018. "The Dog That Almost Barked: What the ACA Repeal Fight Says about the Resilience of the American Welfare State." *Journal of Health Politics, Policy and Law* 43, no. 4: 551–77.

Haggard, Stephan, and Robert R. Kaufman. 2008. *Development, Democracy, and Welfare States: Latin America, East Asia, and Eastern Europe*. Princeton, NJ: Princeton University Press.

Héritier, Adrienne. 1999. *Policy-Making and Diversity in Europe: Escaping Deadlock*. Cambridge: Cambridge University Press.

Howard, Christopher. 1999. *The Hidden Welfare State: Tax Expenditures and Social Policy in the United States*. Princeton, NJ: Princeton University Press.

Katznelson, Ira. 2005. *When Affirmative Action Was White: An Untold History of Racial Inequality in Twentieth-Century America*. New York: Norton.

King, Gary, Robert O. Keohane, and Sidney Verba. 1994. *Designing Social Inquiry: Scientific Inference in Qualitative Research*. Princeton, NJ: Princeton University Press.

Klein, Jennifer. 2003. *For All These Rights: Business, Labor, and the Shaping of America's Public-Private Welfare State*. Princeton, NJ: Princeton University Press.

Lieberman, Evan. 2009. *Boundaries of Contagion: How Ethnic Politics Have Shaped Government Responses to AIDS*. Princeton, NJ: Princeton University Press.

Lieberman, Robert C. 1998. *Shifting the Color Line: Race and the American Welfare State*. Cambridge, MA: Harvard University Press.

Linos, Katerina. 2013. *The Democratic Foundations of Policy Diffusion: How Health, Family, and Employment Laws Spread across Countries*. New York: Oxford University Press.

Lynch, Julia, and Sarah E. Gollust. 2010. "Playing Fair: Fairness Beliefs and Health Policy Preferences in the United States." *Journal of Health Politics, Policy and Law* 35, no. 6: 849–87.

Mahoney, James, and Kathleen Thelen, eds. 2015. *Advances in Comparative-Historical Analysis*. New York: Cambridge University Press.

Maioni, Antonia. 1998. *Parting at the Crossroads: The Emergence of Health Insurance in the United States and Canada*. Princeton, NJ: Princeton University Press.

Marmor, Ted, Richard Freeman, and Kieke Okma. 2005. "Comparative Perspectives and Policy Learning in the World of Health Care." *Journal of Comparative Policy Analysis: Research and Practice* 7, no. 4: 331–48.

Marmor, Theodore R., and Rudolf Klein. 2012. *Politics, Health, and Health Care: Selected Essays*. New Haven, CT: Yale University Press.

Martínez Franzoni, Juliana, and Diego Sánchez-Ancochea. 2018. "Undoing Segmentation? Latin American Health Care Policy during the Economic Boom." *Social Policy and Administration* 52, no. 6: 1181–1200.

Marx, Anthony W. 1998. *Making Race and Nation: A Comparison of South Africa, the United States, and Brazil*. Cambridge: Cambridge University Press.

Maxwell, Angie, and Todd Shields. 2019. *The Long Southern Strategy: How Chasing White Voters in the South Changed American Politics*. New York: Oxford University Press.

Mayes, Rick. 2004. *Universal Coverage: The Elusive Quest for National Health Insurance*. Ann Arbor: University of Michigan Press.

Mettler, Suzanne. 2011. *The Submerged State: How Invisible Government Policies Undermine American Democracy*. Chicago: University of Chicago Press.

Mettler, Suzanne, and Joe Soss. 2004. "The Consequences of Public Policy for Democratic Citizenship: Bridging Policy Studies and Mass Politics." *Perspectives on Politics* 2, no. 1: 55–73.

Morgan, Kimberly J., and Andrea Louise Campbell. 2011. *The Delegated Welfare State: Medicare, Markets, and the Governance of Social Policy*. New York: Oxford University Press.

Morone, James A. 2018. "Health Policy and White Nationalism: Historical Lessons, Disruptive Populism, and Two Parties at a Crossroads." *Journal of Health Politics, Policy and Law* 43, no. 4: 683–706.

Nyhan, Brendan, Eric McGhee, John Sides, Seth Masket, and Steven Greene. 2012. "One Vote Out of Step? The Effects of Salient Roll Call Votes in the 2010 Election." *American Politics Research* 40, no. 5: 844–79.

Oberlander, Jonathan. 2003. *The Political Life of Medicare*. Chicago: University of Chicago Press.

Oberlander, Jonathan. 2016. "Implementing the Affordable Care Act: The Promise and Limits of Health Care Reform." *Journal of Health Politics, Policy and Law* 41, no. 4: 803–26.

Oberlander, Jonathan, and R. Kent Weaver. 2015. "Unraveling from Within? The Affordable Care Act and Self-Undermining Policy Feedbacks." *Forum* 13, no. 1: 37–62.

Obinger, Herbert, Stephan Leibfried, and Francis G. Castles. 2005. "Bypasses to a Social Europe? Lessons from Federal Experience." *Journal of European Public Policy* 23, no. 3: 545–71.

Page, Benjamin I., and Martin Gilens. 2017. *Democracy in America? What Has Gone Wrong and What We Can do About It*. Chicago: University of Chicago Press.

Peterson, Mark A. 2011. "It Was a Different Time: Obama and the Unique Opportunity for Health Care Reform." *Journal of Health Politics, Policy and Law* 36, no. 3: 429–36.

Pierson, Paul. 1996. "The New Politics of the Welfare State." *World Politics* 48, no. 2: 143–79.

Powell, Martin, Daniel Béland, and Alex Waddan. 2018. "The Americanization of the British National Health Service: A Typological Approach." *Health Policy* 122, no. 7: 775–82.

Quadagno, Jill. 2005. *One Nation, Uninsured: Why the US Has No National Health Insurance*. New York: Oxford University Press.

Ragin, Charles C. 1992. "'Casing' and the Process of Social Inquiry." In *What Is a Case? Exploring the Foundations of Social Theory*, edited by Charles C. Ragin and Howard S. Becker, 217–26. New York: Cambridge University Press.

Ragin, Charles C. 2011. *Constructing Social Research: The Unity and Diversity of Method*. Los Angeles: Sage.

Reid, Tom R. 2010. *The Healing of America: A Global Quest for Better, Cheaper, and Fairer Health Care*. New York: Penguin.

Riker, William. 1964. *Federalism: Origins, Operation, Significance*. Boston: Little, Brown.

Saldin, Robert P. 2011. "Healthcare Reform: A Prescription for the 2010 Republican Landslide." *Forum* 8, no. 4: art. 10.

Schneider, Eric C., Dana O. Sarnak, David Squires, and Arnav Shah. 2017. "Mirror, Mirror 2017: International Comparison Reflects Flaws and Opportunities for Better US Health Care." Commonwealth Fund, July 14. www.commonwealthfund.org /publications/fund-reports/2017/jul/mirror-mirror-2017-international-comparison -reflects-flaws-and.

Schoppa, Leonard J. 2006. *Race for the Exits: The Unraveling of Japan's System of Social Protection*. Ithaca, NY: Cornell University Press.

Segatto, Catarina Ianni, and Daniel Béland. 2019. "Federalism and Decision Making in Health Care: The Influence of Subnational Governments in Brazil." *Policy Studies*, June 25. www.tandfonline.com/doi/full/10.1080/01442872.2019.1634187.

Sinclair, Barbara. 2016. *Unorthodox Lawmaking: New Legislative Processes in the US Congress*. Washington, DC: CQ Press.

Sparer, Michael S., Lawrence D. Brown, and Lawrence R. Jacobs. 2009. "Exploring the Concept of Single Payer." *Journal of Health Politics, Policy and Law* 34, no. 4: 447–51.

Stepan, Alfred, and Juan J. Linz. 2011. "Comparative Perspectives on Inequality and the Quality of Democracy in the United States." *Perspectives on Politics* 9, no. 4: 841–56.

Teles, Steven M. 2012. *Kludgeocracy: The American Way of Policy*. Washington, DC: New America Foundation.

Tesler, Michael. 2011. "The Spillover of Racialization Into Health Care: How President Obama Polarized Public Opinion by Racial Attitudes and Race." *American Journal of Political Science* 56, no. 3: 690–704.

Tuohy, Carolyn Hughes. 1999. *Accidental Logics: The Dynamics of Change in the Health Care Arena in the United States, Britain, and Canada*. New York: Oxford University Press.

Tuohy, Carolyn Hughes. 2018. *Remaking Policy: Scale, Pace, and Political Strategy in Health Care Reform*. Toronto: University of Toronto Press.

White, Joseph. 2013. "The 2010 US Health Care Reform: Approaching and Avoiding How Other Countries Finance Health Care." *Health Economics, Policy, and Law* 8, no. 3: 289–315.

Wong, Joseph. 2004. *Healthy Democracies: Welfare Politics in Taiwan and South Korea.* Ithaca, NY: Cornell University Press.

Comparative Perspectives

The Self-Undermining Peril of "Mosaic" Reform Strategies: A Comparative View

Carolyn Hughes Tuohy
University of Toronto

Abstract The American Democratic leadership in the White House and Congress in 2009–10 and the British Conservative/Liberal-Democrat Coalition government in 2010–12 each pursued a strategy of rapidly assembled multiple adjustments to the prevailing policy framework for health care rather than attempting a "big-bang" strategy of sweeping institutional change. Despite their relative modesty, each set of reforms encountered a highly conflictual and tortuous process of legislative passage. Subsequently, the reforms failed to gain broad public acceptance and were variously hobbled (in the United States) and transformed (in the United Kingdom) in the course of implementation. These two cases thus offer some common lessons about the potential and the pitfalls of such complex "mosaic" reforms.

Keywords comparative health policy, health care reform, Affordable Care Act

To paraphrase a clever proverb about history, the politics of health care policy does not repeat itself across national regimes, but on occasion it rhymes. One such rhyming couplet occurred in the United States and Britain at the end of the first decade of the twenty-first century. The American Democratic leadership in the White House and Congress in 2009–10 and the British Conservative/Liberal-Democrat Coalition government in 2010–12 each pursued a strategy of rapidly assembled multiple adjustments to the prevailing system rather than a "big-bang" introduction of a sweeping new institutional regime. Despite their relative modesty, each set of reforms encountered a highly conflictual and tortuous process of legislative passage. Subsequently, the reforms failed to gain broad public acceptance and were variously hobbled (in the United States) and

Journal of Health Politics, Policy and Law, Vol. 45, No. 4, August 2020
DOI 10.1215/03616878-8255601 © 2020 by Duke University Press

transformed (in the United Kingdom) through the implementation process. These two cases thus offer some common lessons about the potential and the pitfalls of such complex "mosaic" reforms.[1]

Mosaic reform strategies represent one of four possible strategic approaches to the scale and pace of policy change (Tuohy 2018). By *scale* I mean the degree and scope of change in the prevailing institutional logic, that is, change in those dimensions of the policy framework that set the balance of influence among key interests, such as the medical profession, the state, and private finance; the mix of instruments, such as hierarchical control, market exchange, and peer persuasion; and the organizing principles defining the function of the state and the obligations and entitlements of citizens. By *pace* I refer to the pace of enactment: are the changes enacted all at once in a single piece of legislation or through successive bills over time? The intersection of scale and pace yields four tendencies: large-fast, large-slow, small-fast, and small-slow. The two principal cases under review here are examples of a strategy of small-fast "mosaic" change (multiple adjustments, enacted as a piece, that do not fundamentally alter the prevailing institutional logic).

The scale and pace of policy change depend on political actors' assessments of their ability to overcome vetoes in the present and over time: how can a reform coalition be built, and how long can it be sustained? In each of the American and British cases reviewed here, the parties in power had strong partisan incentives to move quickly to enact a health care reform that could be presented as a bold achievement. In each case the political leadership judged that it had the necessary institutional and electoral resources to overcome vetoes in the short term but risked losing its position of advantage within a brief time frame. Despite the radical differences in their political institutions and health care systems, each set of political leaders found themselves faced with similar questions of political strategy: how to bridge differences across independent actors within the governments of the day, in order to assemble a winning coalition for a major health care reform within a shrinking time horizon. In so doing they created micro-constituencies of satisfaction with particular elements of the resulting reforms without building understanding or support for the overall package.

American and British Similarities

In 2009 the Democrats under Barack Obama achieved their best electoral results since the Lyndon Johnson's landslide of 1964. They took the

---

1. Each of these cases is much more fully discussed in Tuohy (2018), on which this article draws.

presidency with a solid majority of the popular vote and won control of both chambers of Congress, including for a brief period the razor-thin 60% supermajority in the Senate technically necessary to overcome a Republican filibuster by closing off debate. Obama chose to capitalize on these advantages by tackling a push to universal health insurance coverage that had remained "unfinished business" for the Democrats since the enactment of the targeted Medicare and Medicaid programs (for the elderly and social assistance recipients respectively) under President Johnson in 1965. The window of opportunity was seen to be very tight: Obama and the Democratic leadership initiated the process of drafting health care reform legislation in his first budget within 2 months of his inauguration.

While his position was arguably more favorable than that of any of his predecessors, including even President Johnson (Peterson 2011), Obama still lacked the cohesive coalition necessary for a sweeping institutional change. The independent electoral bases of members of Congress meant that, although the Democratic congressional caucuses were more united than they had been since the beginning of the twentieth century, the leadership still could not rely on the full compliance of their Senate caucus to forestall opposition filibusters. Moreover, the Democrats gained and lost even the nominal cloture threshold in the Senate within 9 months—just long enough for legislation to pass both House and Senate. Reconciling the two bills and completing the process would require yet more bargains and adjustments within the constraints of the process of budget reconciliation requiring only a simple majority.

The result was a layering on of additions to the existing employer-based system: expanding Medicaid to include all those below a set income threshold, establishing state-based health insurance exchanges (later "marketplaces") to facilitate the operation of the individual and small-group markets and to administer income-scaled federal subsidies, and broadening the regulation of private insurance to ban or constrain various underwriting practices. In addition to these three principal components, the reforms were studded with myriad provisions added as the price of securing the votes of individual legislators. Some of the multiple compromises were aimed at luring moderate Republicans; the rest were reached entirely among Democrats after those bipartisan efforts proved fruitless. Among the deals reached were the deferral of some provisions to come into effect over a lengthy 8-year implementation period. These various effective dates were fixed in the legislation—a strategy that would haunt the rollout of the reforms. Despite these various concessions, the legislation attracted no Republican support and triggered an ongoing series of efforts at repeal.

Although such mosaic strategies are less likely to be adopted in the supposedly "veto-free" (Hacker 2004) Westminster system of unified government and party discipline in Britain, they may occur as the result of political calculations. Strategies of scale and pace are determined not by political and institutional conditions themselves but by the ways in which political actors, individually and collectively, read those conditions to assess their prospects for success in the present and over time. In 2010, such calculations led the new Conservative/Liberal-Democrat Coalition toward a mosaic strategy for reform of the National Health Service (NHS). The partners in the Coalition saw the projection of a radical stance as a partisan imperative: they were eager to put a strong and positive face on what otherwise would be seen as a dispiriting election outcome for both parties, in which the Conservatives failed to gain a majority of seats and the Liberal Democrats fell well short of the expectations of only a few months prior. The formation of their unprecedented coalition allowed them to present their partnership as capitalizing on a historic opportunity to embark on new directions. Developing a common agenda, however, required negotiating myriad differences of opinion both between and within the parties. And it would need to be done rapidly: the electoral horizon was even shorter for the two parties in the Coalition than is normal for a Westminster majority government. The parties had agreed to a fixed date for the next election 5 years hence, but they knew they would have to distance themselves from each other increasingly as that deadline approached.

Throughout the process of developing a coalition agreement and a program for government, negotiators at the center of government agreed on a set of reforms to the English NHS. The reforms were essentially an amalgam of Conservative desires for increased competition and greater autonomy within the NHS and Liberal Democrat support for enhanced local authority. They would maintain the logic of the "purchaser/provider split" within the NHS (established two decades earlier by the Thatcher Conservative government and preserved and adapted by subsequent Labour governments) while reconfiguring the "purchasers" essentially to invert the formal relationship between physicians and managers. General practitioners, who had formerly advised local purchasing authorities through professional executive committees, would now form consortia of general practices (subsequently known as clinical commissioning groups) to take over the purchasing function, supported by managerial staff. In addition, numerous other changes were made to the structure and mandate of regulatory and support agencies.

As in the United States, the Coalition government launched the process of health care reform almost immediately and sought to do so with a single piece of legislation. Little over 2 months into its mandate, in July 2010 the government released a white paper fleshing out the reforms—a pace "far faster than any previous health white paper" (Timmins 2012: 15)—and quickly embarked on a period of consultation followed by the introduction of the Health and Social Care Act (HSCA) into the House of Commons in January 2011. However, passage would require numerous compromises during a protracted 14-month legislative process of extraordinary contentiousness, during which the government called an unprecedented "pause" for renewed consultations by a quasi-independent commission, which in turn led the government to support almost 400 substantive amendments (not including minor technical edits) and to adapt its announced approach to implementation (Timmins 2012: 121). The process was fraught with conflict throughout: implacable resistance from the opposition Labour Party was exacerbated by "rebellions" and threatened rebellions in the legislative ranks of the Liberal Democrats in the House of Commons and strong resistance from the more independent members of all parties in the House of Lords. The legislation passed on almost entirely party-line votes in each house, and immediately upon passage the Labour opposition, like the US Republicans, announced its intent to repeal the legislation "at the first opportunity" (Jowit 2012).

Assessing the Politics of Mosaic Reforms in a 10-Year Perspective

What can we learn about the politics of mosaic strategies of policy change by comparing these two cases, not only at the time of their enactment but also in the decade following? The principal observation concerns the self-undermining nature of mosaic strategies, in both process and substance. Both the politics of mosaic strategies and the resultant policy designs have features that leave the reforms open to attack and/or substantial modification in the postenactment period.

Politically, the fast pace of mosaic strategies exacerbates conflict. Enacting changes all at once compresses all veto points into a single episode and forfeits the possibility of dividing the reform process into a series of contests with particular interests while building broader coalitions of support. This phenomenon is especially apparent if we compare the politics of the British coalition reform process with those of the two periods that immediately preceded it: the "big-bang" introduction of the purchaser-provider split under the Thatcher Conservatives in 1990 and the incremental adaptation of that model by Labour from 2000 to 2009. Over that full time span the principles underlying the functional role of the state moved progressively from those of an owner-operator to those closer to a model of a single payer of independent providers. But these phases were marked by very different politics. The fast-paced big bang generated sharp conflict between parties and between the government and affected interests in the health care arena, whereas the incremental Labour phase was a "gradual, step by step process . . . providing little opportunity for a confrontation on the principles underlying the model that finally emerged" (Klein 2013: loc. 7143 of 9801).

Moreover, because they involve coalitions of actors with independent power bases, mosaic strategies typically generate a spectacle of sprawling consultations, inviting continual interventions and feeding public perceptions of incoherence. In addition to the multiple consultations held by the Democratic leadership in Congress and the administration with affected interests, the legislative process for the Affordable Care Act (ACA) comprised 79 hearings involving 181 witnesses in the House and "approximately 100 hearings, roundtables, walkthroughs and other meetings [as well as] 25 consecutive days [of debate] in continuous session" in the Senate (Jost 2017; see also Cannan 2013). Even in a Westminster system, the UK coalition government was forced into an extraordinarily extended and open legislative process, including 50 days of debate plus its midway "pause" for further public consultation.

In terms of policy design, the prospect of losing a position of advantage in the near future that spurs a rapid pace also requires reformers to specify implementation timelines in the original legislation rather than leaving hostages to the fortune of future administrative discretion. This imperative is further complicated when different timelines are attached to different discrete elements of the reforms, often as a result of ad hoc compromises in the process of passage. Both the ACA and the HSCA allowed for phased implementation—in the former case, extending beyond the life of the enacting Congress and the president's first term. In each case, this phased implementation was partly a matter of deliberate design—in the UK case, to allow for the commissioning consortia of general practices to be developed by the numerous local actors involved, and in the US case, to back-end load the costs of the program, given the fiscal constraints of the enactment period. In both cases, however, additional deferrals also resulted from compromises necessary to build the legislative coalition for passage, such as the effective dates for employer mandates, targeted taxes, and payment regimes in the United States, and for the establishment of new bodies and the phasing out of their predecessors in the United Kingdom.

The piecemeal policy design, ad hoc compromises, sprawling negotiations and staggered effective dates characteristic of mosaic reforms set the stage for self-undermining dynamics in the postenactment phase. These dynamics play out in three arenas: the legislature, the implementation process, and public opinion.

The Legislature

Both the ACA and the HSCA encountered vehement opposition from opposition parties that persisted long after the legislation was passed. The multiple attempts, both symbolic and real, of the US Republicans to repeal all or parts of the ACA in the decade following its passage are dealt with elsewhere in this issue. While the Westminster system does not allow for the sort of ongoing repeal attempts mounted by US Republicans, the UK Labour Party took various opportunities to signal its ongoing opposition. When the regulations under the act were published in April 2013, Labour sought to have them annulled by the House of Lords. The regulations easily survived the legislative hurdle, although the government had already tempered them in response to the challenge. In the general elections of 2015, 2017, and 2019, the Labour Party manifesto pledged to repeal the HSCA.

However, in neither the US nor the British case could the opposition accomplish its objective of full legislative repeal. The very point of the fast pace of the reforms was to hardwire them in such a way that they could be repealed only if the opposition could recreate for itself the very conditions that allowed for passage in the first place. In the United Kingdom, this would mean that Labour would have to form a majority government. In the United States, it would mean that the Republicans would not only have to control the White House and both houses of Congress but also be able to forge an internal consensus. Neither British Labour nor the US Republicans were able to clear these bars in the years following passage.

However, the design of the reforms offered other possibilities for opponents, short of outright repeal. Unable to come to an agreement on a legislative package to repeal and replace the ACA despite gaining control of the White House and both houses of Congress, the US Republicans were nonetheless able to defang its most symbolically contentious element, the individual mandate, by repealing the tax penalty for those who did not have health insurance, as part of a broad package of tax reform. The resilience of the ACA reforms was nonetheless demonstrated when, despite fears to the contrary, the individual mandate proved not to be the linchpin whose removal would bring down the entire package but rather to be, in practice, a severable element.[2] British Labour has not yet found itself in a position of advantage similar to the US Republicans. But despite continuing to vow to repeal the HSCA, by the time of the December 2019 election, Labour had narrowed its focus to two symbolically significant elements with modest material effect, pledging specifically to "reinstate the responsibilities of the Secretary of State [for Health] to provide a comprehensive and universal healthcare system" and to "end the requirement on health authorities to put services out to competitive tender" (Labour Party 2019).

The Implementation Process

The piecemeal nature of mosaic reforms can be both a strength and a liability, offering opportunities for various political actors to either chip away at or adapt them in the implementation process. Consider first the opportunities for opponents. The multiple disjointed elements of mosaic reforms are likely to vary in their vulnerability to legal challenge and administrative discretion in implementation. They therefore provide a number of footholds for those who would seek to overturn or modify the reforms even without building the coalition that would be necessary for broad legislative change. These opportunities are multiplied to the extent that political institutions allow for "venue shifting" as quintessentially afforded by the checks and balances and federal division of powers in the American political system, in contrast to the more unified British Westminster model. Republican opponents of the ACA were able to use the courts and state governments to frustrate or constrain some of its aspects, notably the expansion of Medicaid. State refusals to establish health insurance exchanges in all or part also resulted in a greater federal role in that aspect of the reforms by default than had been envisaged at the outset.

In the United Kingdom, the piecemeal nature of the HSCA reforms allowed them to be recombined in implementation without legislative change, to an effect quite different than what the foundational model of the "purchaser/provider split" would imply. A new chief executive of NHS England, appointed in 2014, moved progressively to reintegrate activities that had been separated in the name of increased autonomy and choice.

---

2. The severability of the universal mandate as a matter of law nonetheless continued to be litigated.

New models of integrated care that would blur the distinction between purchasing and provision functions have been promoted, and new structures and processes that effectively reintegrate executive functions at both central and regional levels have been put in place—all through administrative action.

A final vulnerability of mosaic reform strategies stems from their characteristic staggering of the effective dates of various elements. In theory an attenuated implementation timetable can allow for the development of technological and other capacity before reforms come onstream. But when implementation dates are specified in the legislation up front, implementers are tied to a fixed timeline whether or not capacity development has proceeded as anticipated, thus providing opportunities for opponents to seize upon and exacerbate administrative difficulties. Because of their nature as packages of elements that are more the result of hasty compromises than of policy design, mosaic strategies are particularly vulnerable to such problems. This was particularly apparent in implementing the ACA—most notoriously in the case of the problem-ridden launch of the federal enrolment platform, HeathCare.gov, in October 2013, but also when the effective dates for a variety of provisions arrived before those at whom they were targeted (e.g., employers and insurers) had developed the capacity to comply. Unable to adapt the legislation itself in the polarized partisan Congress, the Obama administration controversially took administrative action on more than 20 occasions between January 2013 and March 2015 to provide "significant" delays, extensions, exemptions, provisions for retroactive payments, and other deviations from the strict provisions of the ACA in order to smooth its implementation (Redhead and Kinzer 2015).

Tactical choices can nonetheless mitigate such problems. Faced with deferred effective dates, the British Coalition government put in place a number of the new entities in "shadow" form to operate de facto through various forms of delegation, to ready them in advance of the dates at which the legislation would provide them with de jure authority. Conversely, some legacy bodies were retained longer than anticipated, as administrative support while the new or transforming entities were developing capacity.

Public Opinion

Because mosaic reforms touch multiple parts of the system yet lack a coherent overall frame, they are vulnerable to being portrayed as both chaotic and overweening, generating and perpetuating public confusion

Table 1 Support for Healthcare Reform Legislation One Month Before Passage, US 2010 and UK 2012, by Party Affiliation

	US February 2010[1]				UK February 2012[2]			
	Democrat	Independent	Republican	All	Conservative	Liberal Democrat	Labour	All
Support	**70**	39	14	43	39	9	3	14
Oppose	16	**45**	**74**	43	19	**50**	**76**	48
Don't know	14	16	12	15	**42**	41	21	38

1. "As of right now, do you generally support or generally oppose the health care proposals being discussed in Congress?" (Kaiser Family Foundation 2010).
2. "The government's proposed reforms of the National Health Service are currently going through Parliament. From what you have seen or heard about them, do you support or oppose the government's NHS reforms?" (YouGov 2012).

and hostility. In the case of both the ACA and the HSCA, public reaction to the legislation divided along partisan lines. In the United Kingdom sheer confusion dominated that partisan effect, whereas in the United States voters appeared to take their cues from their parties in forming their views. Table 1 shows opinion in each of the two countries 1 month before passage of the legislation. In the United Kingdom, partisan opposition was most sharply apparent among Labour voters, whereas supporters of the two parties in the governing coalition, and especially the Liberal Democrats, were more divided and much more likely than Labour voters to register a "don't know" response. In part this may be because neither the Conservatives nor the Liberal Democrats had given any signal in their election manifestos that they would enter into coalition, much less embark on major reform to the NHS, whereas American Democratic voters had been in no doubt that health care reform would figure prominently on the Democratic agenda. Notwithstanding their differences regarding the merits of the legislation itself, however, Democrats, Republicans, and Independents in the United States were alike in their propensity to see the politics of its passage as less about "fundamental disagreements on what would be the right policy for the country" than about "both sides playing politics with the issue" (Kaiser Family Foundation 2010).

What is more interesting from a decade-long perspective is the extent to which these attitudes persisted. In part, this persistence may have been fed by difficulties and contention in rolling out the reforms as discussed above, reinforcing the perception of incoherence. In the United States, the persistence of the partisan divide in public opinion has been well documented, including elsewhere in this issue. In the United Kingdom, there is evidence of a similar phenomenon. The sharp decline in satisfaction with "the way in which the NHS runs nowadays" that coincided with the parliamentary debates over the reforms in 2011 reversed a 10-year trajectory of increasing satisfaction and marked the onset of a pattern of fluctuation around a general declining trend (Robertson et al. 2019: 6). Partisan differences continued: in 2018, Conservatives were more likely to be satisfied; Labour supporters, less so. Evidence is mixed as to the impact of the reforms themselves on public satisfaction, at a time when the coalition and subsequent Conservative governments were also constraining rates of annual increases in NHS funding after a decade of funding increases under Labour. Initially the new austerity appeared not to trigger strong opposition: a majority of respondents in the 2014 British Social Attitudes survey supported the current level of spending, with only about a third arguing that the government should "spend more" (Curtice and Ormston 2015). Later, however, respondents to the survey from 2015 to 2018 were consistently more likely to cite insufficient government spending than to cite "government reforms" as a cause for dissatisfaction (at about 40–50% and 20–30%, respectively) (Robertson et al. 2019: 15).

A Within-Country Comparison

The ACA is not the only case of a mosaic strategy in the history of American health care reform. Given the multiple veto points inherent in the US political system, it is perhaps not surprising that the very founding of the modern US health care state—the Medicare/Medicaid legislation of 1965—required a mosaic strategy, producing the original "three-layer cake" of additions to the employer-based model as disparate proposals for physician and hospital services for the elderly and health care services for low-income families were amalgamated to attract a winning coalition. This process of negotiation yielded "a model of unintended consequences [that] . . . incorporated features that no one had fully foreseen" (Marmor 2000: 58–59).

The parallels and differences between Medicare/Medicaid and the ACA suggest some qualification of our propositions about the dynamics of mosaic reforms. Each reform package was born in open legislative conflict as well as behind-the-sciences negotiations. The ACA process brokered factionalism within the Democratic Party to yield a purely Democratic result against unanimous Republican opposition; the Medicare/Medicaid process deeply divided the Democratic Party, even as it attracted some

Republican support. These conflicts played out in public view as various bills ran the legislative gauntlet (Marmor 2000: 46–61). Moreover, although the Medicare/Medicaid package was a relatively more elegant result than the rather jumbled ACA, even it was a pastiche of competing proposals.

In both cases, reformers focused on what was at the time a relatively small segment of the private insurance market and on the medically indigent. Medicare and Medicaid targeted the elderly and social assistance recipients, respectively. The ACA was aimed at covering those uninsured or underinsured under either public programs or private insurance. In each case the degree of institutional change within these segments was significant. Although Medicare/Medicaid built on the established Social Security model, the extension of that model to health care represented a significant increase in the weight and a change in the role of the state. Similarly, by expanding Medicaid the ACA built on an established program but substantially increased its redistributive effect, and the establishment of health care marketplaces introduced a significant innovation in the regulatory role of the state.

The *scope* of the two sets of reforms varied, however, in ways that had important implications for their future dynamics. While Medicare imposed an obligation on most employers and workers to contribute to Part A of the program, those contributions built on the well-accepted Social Security program. And while Medicare and Medicaid potentially affected all physicians and hospitals, the two programs essentially added another (public) payer to the mix of private payers to which those providers were accustomed, and those relationships with other payers were left alone. No grand accommodation, such as that binding the medical profession and the state into exclusive or near-exclusive relationships in the founding models of the health care state in Canada and the United Kingdom, was brought about. Meanwhile, employer-based coverage for the bulk of the population, as well as the norms and commercial reach of the private insurance industry, were left intact.[3]

In contrast to this delimited mosaic, the ACA made small adjustments to the rules of the game that touched almost all actors in the health arena. In addition to the changes to Medicaid and to the individual and small-group

3. There is also a significant tactical difference between the Johnson and Obama mosaics. Perhaps owing to Johnson's famous aversion to any delay that would allow opposition to build (Blumenthal and Morone 2010: 190), legislative compromises did not include the deferral of effective dates of various provisions. With Johnson's personal involvement, implementation proceeded rapidly (Blumenthal and Morone 2010: 198; Ball and Hess 2001: 8–9), in contrast to the staggered ACA implementation discussed above.

insurance market, the reforms addressed underwriting practices and profit margins of private insurers more broadly, in addition to many other provisions added to the legislation as the price of passage. The changes thus affected, at the margins, not only all providers of covered services but also all insurers and many employers. (In this respect the ACA reforms were more similar to the HSCA reforms in England. Although the latter effectively accelerated changes already under way under the previous Labour government, the organizational changes simultaneously affected all purchasers and providers of NHS services. In both the ACA and the HSCA cases, the pervasiveness of the changes conveyed the impression of a gargantuan reform, while the complexity and incoherence of the package made it difficult for proponents to build support by communicating its overall purpose and intended benefits.)

The postpassage politics of the two American sets of reforms were starkly different. There is no parallel in the Medicare/Medicaid case to the unrelenting opposition of Republicans to the ACA and their ongoing attempts at repeal and constitutional challenge (Patashnik and Oberlander 2018: 663). Nor did public support decline over the course of the Medicare/Medicaid legislative debate and thereafter, in further contrast to experience with the ACA (Blendon and Benson 2001: 35–36). Medicare and Medicaid have not only persisted but also expanded on balance over time, in part because of demographic change, but also as a matter of deliberate policy choices.

The contrasts between these two American cases suggest some further nuance to the propositions offered here about the postenactment dynamics of mosaic reforms. Mosaics largely confined to a segment of the health care arena may prove more durable than those whose effects are more widespread. Conversely, multiple small changes that are spread across the arena exacerbate the problem of conveying the coherence and point of the reforms and provide multiple footholds for opposition. In short, the scope of change may be at least as important for postenactment politics as is its degree. Our few cases are not sufficient to explore this hypothesis further, but they raise questions for further research.

A final caveat: any comparison of strategies of scale and pace in policy change, across or within nations, needs to situate those cases in their historical-institutional context more fully than space allows here (Tuohy 2018). In the American context, comparisons between the 1960s and 2010s are complicated not only by increasing partisan polarization over that period but also by the fact that Medicare and Medicaid have become part of the historical-institutional context in which the ACA played out (Patashnik and Oberlander 2018). Indeed, it can be argued that the feedback effects of those two programs have been to reinforce the structure of the programs themselves while making it more politically difficult to adopt broader-based designs. Nonetheless, similarities in political dynamics of mosaic strategic across historical-institutional contexts as different as the United States and the United Kingdom in the early twenty-first century suggest that choices of scale and pace have significant effects at the margin.

A mosaic strategy may well be a reasonable choice in political circumstances such as those confronting the framers of the ACA. Other political actors facing analogous circumstances would nonetheless be well advised to be alert to the potentially self-undermining properties of such strategies and to consider how they can be mitigated.

■ ■ ■

Carolyn Hughes Tuohy is professor emeritus of political science and a distinguished fellow in the Munk School of Global Affairs and Public Policy at the University of Toronto. She specializes in comparative public policy, with an emphasis on social policy. She is the author of four books, most recently *Remaking Policy: Scale, Pace, and Political Strategy in Health Care Reform* (2018), as well as four coedited books and numerous journal articles and book chapters on health and social policy, professional regulation, and comparative approaches in public policy. She is a Fellow of the Royal Society of Canada.
c.tuohy@utoronto.ca

References

Ball, Robert M., and Arthur E. Hess. 2001. "Dialogue on Implementing Medicare." In *Reflections on Implementing Medicare*, edited by Michael G. Gluck and Virginia Reno, 1–30. Washington, DC: National Academy of Social Insurance.

Blendon, Robert J., and John M. Benson. 2001. "Americans' Views on Health Policy: A Fifty-Year Historical Perspective." *Health Affairs* 20, no. 2: 33–46.

Blumenthal, David, and James A. Morone. 2010. *The Heart of Power: Health and Politics in the Oval Office*. Berkeley: University of California Press.

Cannan, John. 2013. "A Legislative History of the Affordable Care Act: How Legislative Procedure Shapes Legislative History." *Law Library Journal* 105, no. 2: 131–73.

Curtice, John, and Rachel Ormston. 2015. "Key Findings: The Verdict on Five Years of Coalition Government." British Social Attitudes, NatCen Social Research,

32 ed. www.bsa.natcen.ac.uk/latest-report/british-social-attitudes-32/key-findings
/introduction.aspx (accessed February 12, 2020).

Hacker, Jacob. 2004. "Dismantling the Health Care State? Political Institutions, Public
Policies, and the Comparative Politics of Health Reform." *British Journal of
Political Science* 34, no. 4: 693–724.

Jost, Timothy. 2017. "Examining the House Republican ACA Repeal and Replace
Legislation." *Health Affairs Blog*, March 7. healthaffairs.org/blog/2017/03/07
/examining-the-house-republican-aca-repeal-and-replace-legislation/.

Jowit, Juliette. 2012. "NHS Reform: Health and Social Care Bill Passes Its Final
Hurdle." *Guardian*, March 20. www.theguardian.com/politics/2012/mar/20/nhs
-reform-health-bill-passes-vote.

Kaiser Family Foundation. 2010. "Kaiser Health Tracking Poll—February 2010."
February 1. www.kff.org/health-reform/poll-finding/kaiser-health-tracking-poll
-february-2010/.

Klein, Rudolf. 2013. *The New Politics of the NHS*. 7th ed. Abington, UK: Radcliffe.
Kindle Edition.

Labour Party. 2019. "Manifesto: Rebuild Our Public Services." labour.org.uk
/manifesto/rebuild-our-public-services/ (accessed February 7, 2020).

Marmor, Theodore R. 2000. *The Politics of Medicare*. 2nd ed. New York: Aldine de
Gruyter.

Patashnik, Eric M., and Jonathan Oberlander. 2018. "After Defeat: Conservative
Postenactment Opposition to the ACA in Historical-Institutional Perspective."
Journal of Health Politics, Policy and Law 43, no. 4: 651–82.

Peterson, Mark A. 2011. "It Was a Different Time: Obama and the Unique Opportunity
for Health Care Reform." *Journal of Health Politics, Policy and Law* 36, no. 3:
429–36.

Redhead, C. Stephen, and Janet Kinzer. 2015. "Implementing the Affordable Care
Act: Delays, Extensions, and Other Actions Taken by the Administration." Congressional Research Service, March 3. fas.org/sgp/crs/misc/R43474.pdf.

Robertson, Ruth, John Appleby, Harry Evans, and Nina Hemmings. 2019. "Public
Satisfaction with the NHS and Social Care in 2018: Results from the British Social
Attitudes Survey." King's Fund, March 7. www.kingsfund.org.uk/publications
/public-satisfaction-nhs-social-care-2018.

Timmins, Nicholas. 2012. *Never Again? The Story of the Health and Social Care Act,
2012*. London: Institute for Government and King's Fund.

Tuohy, Carolyn Hughes. 2018. *Remaking Policy: Scale, Pace, and Political Strategy
in Health Care Reform*. Toronto: University of Toronto Press.

YouGov. 2012. "YouGov/*Sunday Times* Survey Results." cdn.yougov.com/cumulus_
uploads/document/eqllmvsaav/YG-Archives-Pol-ST-results-24-260212.pdf (accessed February 7, 2020).

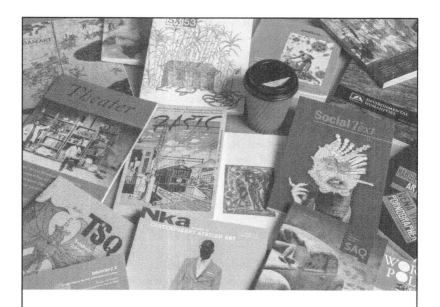

Keep up to date on new scholarship

Issue alerts are a great way to stay current on all the cutting-edge scholarship from your favorite Duke University Press journals. This free service delivers tables of contents directly to your inbox, informing you of the latest groundbreaking work as soon as it is published.

To sign up for issue alerts:

1. Visit **dukeu.press/register** and register for an account. You do not need to provide a customer number.

2. After registering, visit **dukeu.press/alerts**.

3. Go to "Latest Issue Alerts" and click on "Add Alerts."

4. Select as many publications as you would like from the pop-up window and click "Add Alerts."

read.dukeupress.edu/journals

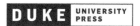

Printed and bound by CPI Group (UK) Ltd, Croydon, CR0 4YY

13/04/2025

14656479-0005